Alternative Therapy Sequel: 4

NOTES ON SPAGYRICS

By

Prof. Dr. Debasish Kundu

M.D.H., F.F.Hom, F.I.H.M.S., Ph.D.(U.S.A.), D.Sc. (Colombo)

Originals

Delhi

First Edition 1999

Published by:

International Holistic Medical Society P.O.Box 66005,
Stockton,CA 95206,USA

Second Revised Edition 2017

ISBN 13: 978-81-8454-170-0
ISBN 10: 81-8454-170-8

Published By

Originals

A-6, Second Floor, Nimri Commercial Centre,
Ashok Vihar Phase-4, Delhi - 110 052 (India)
Tel.: +91 11 2730 2453 Fax: 011 4706 1936
website: www.Lppindia.com e-mail: info@Lppindia.com

Printed At

D K Fine Art Press P Ltd.
Delhi-110052

PRINTED IN INDIA

Dedication

In the Loving Memory of

My Mother Shefalika Kundu

To my Spiritual Teacher

Tantracharya Indrajit Banerjee

Prof. Dr. Debasish Kundu

M.D.H., F.F.Hom, F.I.H.M.S., Ph.D.(U.S.A.), D.Sc.(Colombo)

Fellow of International Holistic Medical Society, CA, U.S.A.
Fellow of Foundation of Homeopathy, MO, U.S.A.
Fellow of World E.Homeopathy System of Medical Council, Hong Kong
Faculty, International Holistic Medical Society, CA, U.S.A.
Faculty, Association of Independent Natural Science Schools Colleges, Professions & Arts, MO, U.S.A.
Vice-President, American Nutritional Medical Association, CA, U.S.A.
Foreign Bureau Chief (India), Holistic Medical Hylite International, CA, U.S.A.
Visiting Professor, Khulna Homeopathic Medical College & Hospital, Khulna, Bangladesh
Ex-Director General, Mooreland University, U.S.A.
Former Adjunct. Faculty & Associate Professor, Department of Human Behavior, Newport University, U.S.A.
Editor In Chief, International Journal of Homeopathy & Natural Medicines, USA
Editor in Chief, The Internet Journal of Herbal and Plant Medicine, USA

Author,
Diseases of Women,
Natural Medicines,
A Clinical Treatise on Cancer,
Aids & Homeopathy,
Pharmacodynamics,
Aids & Your Sex Life,
Aids & Homeopathy,
Essentials of Acupuncture,
Materia Medica for the New Age Man, etc.
Recipient, Royal Assyrian Order of Merit (OIUCM, 1993)
Laureate, United Nations Dag Hammarskjold Award for Medicine (1995)
Recipient, Special Achievement Award, International Conference on E. Omeopatia, Poretta Terme, Bologna, Italy (2008)

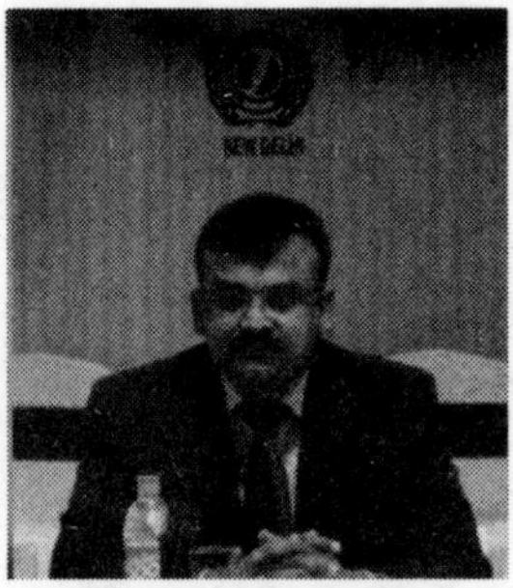

Foreword

I am pleased to have the opportunity to write foreword for the book of Notes on Spagyrics which is written by Dr. Debasish Kundu for ADEH students. Because I have a dream for all my Electro Homoeopathic practitioners that one day they must get an official Certificate from any Government Agency and I am happy to say that Maharashtra is the First State in India to offer an Official Electro Homoeopathy Certificate which is being awarded by the Government Agency. Also I have some friends who helped me to fulfill my dream to introduce a Government recognised ADVANCE DIPLOMA IN ELECTRO HOMOEOPATHY (ADEH) course in Maharashtra.

When word comes "ADVANCED" means something new and scientific, so while reading the contents of the book, I found something new and advanced. Since long time Dr. Kundu is writing books on different subjects which are very easy to understand and rich in contents, so I believe this book will help all the Students, Practitioners & Lovers of Electro-Homoeopathy besides students in perusing ADEH examination which contains the study material mentioned in Syllabus by MSBVE, Mumbai. This entire course material will help to improve the knowledge in Electro Homoeopathy subject.

Dr. Trideep Guha
BPTH, MD (ECH) MBA, Ph.D., MRCE (USA)
Chairman
Educational & Medical/Paramedical Council of India
Executive Member:
Paramedical Syllabus Committee,
MSBVEE, Mumbai (Govt. of Maharashtra)

Email id
drtrideep.g@gmail.com, empci@hotmail.com
Visit us at :
www.empci.com

Published By

Originals

A-6, Second Floor, Nimri Commercial Centre,
Ashok Vihar Phase-4, Delhi - 110 052 (India)
Tel.: +91 11 2730 2453 Fax: 011 4706 1936
Website: www.Lppindia.com
e-mail: info@Lppindia.com

In Association with

ADEH PRACTISIONERS ASSOCIATION MAHARASHTRA

N-123, Second floor, Infront of Devanjali flats,
Reshimbag, City & District : Nagpur
State : Maharashtra Country : INDIA
Phone : +91-712-2700606, +91-712-2700651, +91-712-2700777

Note to the Readers:

Every possible effort has been made to ensure that the information contained in this book is accurate and the author cannot accept responsibility for any errors or omissions, however caused.

No responsibility for loss or damage occasioned to any person acting, or refraining from action, as a result of the material in this publication can be accepted by the author. The author is not associated with any website or product mentioned in the book. The contents of this work are intended to further general scientific research, understanding and discussion only. Readers should consult with a specialist where appropriate.

Every effort has been made to trace the owners of copyright material used in this book, if any. The author and the publisher will be grateful for any omission brought to their notice for acknowledgement in the future editions of the book.

Preface

"Alchemy is no mere fantasy, but a philosophy
applied to the world,
to the elements, to the animals,
and to man himself,"

W.B. Yeats

According to legend, the science of spiritual liberation known as Alchemy was imparted to humanity as a gift from the gods who descended from the heavens around the time of Atlantis and Lemuria some thirteen thousand years ago. The knowledge then made its way through Sumeria now modern day Iraq, considered one of the birth-places of civilization. The knowledge continues through India, Egypt, China, South America, Israel, Europe, and North America. This cosmic drama spans the length of recorded history up to the present day and addresses the deepest questions of life. This gift of spiritual technology is for the purpose of embodied liberation of the human soul where by ones evolutionary soul growth is accelerated to completion within one lifetime. The illusion of individual separation gives way to unity with the transcendent through the transformation of conscious awareness and liberation of the soul from the cycle of birth and death. The transmigration of the soul from incarnation to incarnation reaches completion and fulfillment. This is also known as illumination, enlightenment, transfiguration, ascension, or God realization.

Alchemy preceded modern chemistry. It began in Asia, Egypt, Persia, and Mesopotamia. There are records of alchemists in Alexandria around 300 BC. From there it spread to India, China and to Europe. Alchemists made many important discoveries and developed equipment and procedures that we still use today. They contributed to metallurgy, dyeing, glass making, and medicine. Their work advanced our knowledge of the physical world.

In the Middle Ages, court alchemists worked to transmute base metals into gold to provide wealth for their sponsors. They often conducted their experiments in secret and kept their records using symbols to represent chemical ingredients. As a result of this, alchemy is often thought of as mysticism, magic, or fraud. Materials included in this text are the modules consist of exclusive texts, manuals, drawings, dictionary and sketches besides information on ingredients and planetary herbs.

I believe this text will serve as a veritable guide for the truth seekers.

Dr. Debasish Kundu

Contents

Contents

1
Introduction

Spagyric is a name given to the production of herbal medicines using alchemical procedures. Originated from Greek: Spao, to tear open, + ageiro, to collect. It is a term coined by Paracelsus. These procedures involve fermentation, distillation and the extraction of mineral components from the ash of the plant. These processes were in use in medieval alchemy generally for the separation and purification of metals from ores, and salts from brines and other aqueous solutions.

Nagarjuna an Indian metallurgist and alchemist, born at Fort Daihak near Somnath in Gujarat in 931. He wrote the very first treatise Rasaratnakara that deals with alchemical preparations.

Spagyric medicine is ancient natural medicine the has undergone 500 years of trial, research and practice. Paracelsus the famous Swiss physician, Philosopher and alchemist is regarded as the founder of spagyric, but it was almost forgotten until the 19th century.

Dating from thee times of Paracelsus, the terms spagyric and spagyrism are derived from the Greek verbs "span (to seperate) and ageirein (to unify)". They designate the art of creating medications of enhanced efficacy by performing the two fundamental alchemical operations. The valuable portions are first separated from those which are impure processed and subsequently reunited to yield an improved medicinal form (Axel Helmstadter, 1990). The source materials of spagyric medicines are exclusively from botanical origin. Depending upon the manufacturing process, differentiation is made among spagyrism according to Krauss.

The preparation of spagyric essences is not always the same. There is no uniform method in the preparation as seen in homeopathy and even the Philosophy may vary among the systems of spagyric methods. Even though there are similarities in homeopathy and spagyrics, the roots of both systems being too different. The effectiveness of both preparations depend mainly on the therapist. This decides whether the use of any of the medicines will have the most beneficial effect or not. Spagyric includes alchemistic principles, rooting in ancient Egypt. In Europe, Paracelsus has been an important advocate of Spagyric. Homeopathy came much later. Spagyric is derived from "span" = to separate, and "ageirein" = to combine. Through various processes in essence-preparation both is achieved. In the remedy, larger organic molecules are not found anymore. So, poisoning by substances can not take place, even if poisonous plants are used.

The two active principles in a human being are energy and matter, energy sustains matter, just as air supplies the body with life. One's energetic state of being directly correlates with the quality of form, and though all beings are qualitatively the same primordial substance, quantitatively they differ. Evolve to embody the highest incarnate state a human being can achieve. But, living energy is not fixed, all effects have multiple influences, in a complex interrelationship with one-another, reflecting that of all living things, plants, minerals, metals, animals, and human beings. spagyrism offers an opportunity not only for health, specifically targeting the issue, or general support, but an opportunity to interact with living Intelligences constitutionally.

The three constituents of a balanced being are Salt, Mercury, and Sulfur. Salt is the physical body, the container of form binding the other principles together, in plants/herbs it resides in the mineral components, cellular structure, and hard tissues, alcohol and fermentation products, essential oils, and resins. Mercury is the emotional body, and the life-force energy which animates and mediates life (spirit). All sensuality relies on vital life-force energy inherent in all existence, thus the instinct for Self-preservation, not of the identity or ego, but the real intelligence, intrinsic and instinctual. Mercury, the Prima Materia (Primary or Primordial Substance), is the elixir of life ("Water of Life"; Arabic "exixer"). One must focus on the strength of one's life-force energy, it determines health. Mercurial life-force energy or Veriditas mediates between life-force energy and matter; this soma/haoma/manna is a law, the function of life or the sap of a living plant, the Fire of Tantra. The highest level of Al-Iksirs are called Magisteries. Sulfur, the mental body or soul, is the highest state to work on, effecting all cloudy states, this work is considered truly magical.

Alchemy is based on the belief that there are four basic elements: fire, air, earth and water, and three essentials: salt, sulphur and mercury. Great symbolic and metaphysical systems have been built from these seven pillars of alchemy.

The spagyric medicines are prepared by a specific process called the 'cohobation' which was introduced by Dr. Theoparastus Von Honheim (Paracelsus) in which the living energies of the plant remain in the essences so obtained. Spagyric remedies were originally created by fermenting parts of wild herbs. This process produced concentrated aromatic solutions that were extracted and separated from the plant matter. After fermentation, the plant material was distilled, and the remainder dried and burned. The ashes were extracted and purified via distillation and crystallized, then recombined with the concentrated solution. As a result, the finished spagyric essence contained the mineral constituent parts of the plant which preserves the vital energies of the plant stored up in the essences so obtained. Because of the distillation process Spagyric medicines retain the electrolyte properties of the plants and this is critical to the healing process.

Spagyrics balances any imbalance in these three constituents. Each constituent, Salt, Mercury, and Sulfur, has one of seven possible celestial archetypes or planetary rulerships, determined by day and time of birth (constitution) showing the planetary energies one has the greatest need for, and which are most likely to become imbalanced, causing the degeneration (from which disease stems).

Our Phyto-nucleus Spagyric essences contain:

Organic compounds of low molecular substances (organic chemistry) and Mineral salts and oligo elements (inorganic chemistry), components of the organism representing between 4-5% of the human body weight. Mineral salts are essential to its proper operation, ensuring normal growth and maintenance of bones and teeth, blood clotting and muscular contraction. Trace elements can only be found in very small quantities in the organism; they take part in numerous metabolic reactions, acting as catalysts. Spagyric medicines due to their unique method of preparation are rich in micronutrients and trace elements, which help defend the body against the debilitating effects of chelation or salt hunger, in addition, these remedies promote the excretion of biologically incompatible electromagnetic frequencies and toxic substances from the human organism, including those caused by malnutrition and exposure to sources of electromagnetic fields. Most plants used to produce Spagyric essences are very rich in minerals that are very well absorbed by the body. It is the essence of the life force energy present in the organism which revives our cells and prevents further deterioration of each cell continuously reviving them.

Spagyric medicine, and alchemical methodology, recognizes that the attunement of one's energy-field, mind, heart, and physical body, is integral, and that all must be synergistically phase-synced, aligned, for optimal health.

Spagyrics is a blend of spirituality, philosophy and science. Science states that through matter life was created: in alchemy, it was life that created matter; everything was created from one source of matter and that matter created the three Essentials: Mercury, Sulphur and Salt. But it has nothing to do either with the mercury or sulphur or even salt. Some opined that alchemy is the psychological aspects in life, inner alchemy and sexual alchemy. But the older scriptures described alchemy in a way that would almost be considered early chemistry.

Most traditional healing practices are based on intuitive principles of diseases involving the imbalance of elemental qualities. In the middle ages, alchemists worked to trans- mute base metals into gold and conducted their experiments in secret and kept their records using symbols to represent ingredients. As a result, alchemy was regarded as mysticism, black magic or fraud. The alchemical paintings added much mystery to this stigma.

The magical substance that was to transmute metals, to be the universal panacea and to serve as the key to immortality, was called the philosopher's stone. Alchemy is based on the belief that there are four basic elements: fire, air, earth and water, and three essentials: salt, sulphur and mercury. Great symbolic and metaphysical systems have been built from these seven pillars of alchemy.

2

History of Alchemy

Extraction Technologies for medicinal aromatic plants in Indian subcontinent are historically established nearly 3000 years ago for healing the mankind. About 2500 years ago Ayurvedic system of medicine spread to the country followed by Siddha from south India, Unani from Arabia and acupuncture from China. The Ayurveda and traditional system of medicine which uses extracts of many species of flora of the country mainly depend on traditional technologies for their primary health care needs.

Ancient Chinese and Egyptian occult literature are said to be the foundation upon which alchemy is based. Alchemy was very popular in mediaeval Europe where one of the most sacred books of the al-chemists was allegedly written by the Egyptian god Thoth, known as Hermes Trismegistus (Hermes, the thrice-great, was the Greek god who served as a messenger and delivered the souls of the dead to Hades.) In 1455, a manuscript entitled Corpus Hermeticum began circulating in Florence, Italy. It was allegedly a compilation of the alchemical, astrological and magical knowledge of the Egyptian god. However, it is now known that the work was of European origin and dates from somewhat after the time Thoth prospered. The work is full of magic spells and incantations and other useless occult notions. Today, the transmutation motif is largely ignored, while the transcendence and medical motifs are still going strong in areas such as homeopathy and aromatherapy. Many modern alchemists combine their occult art with astrology, acupuncture, hypnosis and a wide variety of New Age spiritual quests. Unlike modern chemistry, which grew out of alchemy, the ancient art is heavily spiritual.

Alchemists may have been the first ones to try out their ideas by devising experiments, but because of their intensely metaphysical purposes and beliefs, alchemists did not develop modern scientific methods. Alchemy never separated itself from the supernatural, the magical and the superstitious. Perhaps that is why it is still popular, even though it has accomplished practically nothing of lasting value. Alchemists never transmuted metals, never found a panacea, and never discovered the fountain of youth. Some alchemists did make contributions to the advancement of knowledge, however. For example, Paracelsus introduced the concept of disease to medicine. He rejected the notion that disease is a matter of imbalance or disharmony in the body, even though modern alchemists favour this view. Instead, Paracelsus maintained that agents outside of the body, which attack it, cause disease. He recommended various chemicals to fight disease. Several authorities opined that since alchemy was referred to at that time as "black art" or "witchcraft", some medical reformers like Hahnemann simply avoided making any direct references to alchemy. However, we know alchemy is the mother of modern chemistry and in both ayurveda and homeopathy some alchemical methods are incorporated, as in making Rasasindura in ayurveda and Hepar sulph in homeopathy.

It was not until the 1970s that historians of science began to accept alchemy as a valid contributor to seventeenth-century medicine. Frances Yates was the first historian to explore the medical world of the alchemist in her book, The Rosicrucian Enlightenment (1979). In it, she opined that alchemy was wholly mystical, showing instead that during the sixteenth and seventeenth centuries numerous alchemists developed highly advanced scientific theories, many of which greatly affected the European medical community.

Philosophers and historians of pharmacy regard it as a science and philosophy, Alchemy provided the beginnings of chemistry, and certainly helped to develop the apparatus of chemistry. It is part of the history of science, which is the history of human interaction with nature, and humanity's attempts to harness the power of nature for very human needs and wants.

Alchemists acted on the idea that nature had secrets to give and that they could be revealed through laboratory examination and experimentation. While their knowledge was limited regarding the properties of nature, nonetheless, the work of the alchemists provided the basis of modern laboratory techniques, and they did indeed discover many of nature's secrets. Their dogged pursuit for the elixir of life is not so different from modern chemists and natural products researchers who are similarly searching for that one great find which will cure all ills.

Was alchemy magic? Was "magic" used in the processes of alchemy? That question remains. One answer to that question is that "magic" is anything that cannot yet be explained through science and/or reason. Certainly, in seeking the secrets of nature, some alchemists were searching for a greater connection to "God," to the spirit moving the world. There was also a great deal of astrology at play in the work of alchemy, as was ritual in the laboratory processes. Laboratories were laid out based on cosmic conjunctions and designed as if in a temple. Some would argue that this was "magic." Particularly after the 14th century, Alchemy became more closely associated with magic. Clergymen were forbidden to practice it, by and large, so it was taken up by laymen. The era of witchhunts was well under way, and alchemists were often viewed as magicians and sorcerers who were worthy of persecution for their activities. Complicating matters were those, like Heinrich Cornelius Agrippa, who believed they were wizards who could call forth spirits and other mystical forces to their service. Without a doubt, there were many false practitioners of alchemy whose main goal was the transmutation of base metal into gold who were using something like "hocus pocus" in their sleight-of-hand machinations to fool the public. Nevertheless, a belief in something at work that was not the result of human action was essential, especially early on.

Not until Paracelsus in the 16th century was alchemy pulled away from the stigma of "magic" when he, among others, began promoting the experimental aspects of it over the philosophical and spiritual. Many later practitioners of the 17th and 18th centuries were well-known scientists with solid reputations and who are revered to this day for their many other accomplishments. Alchemy was just one of many scientific pursuits for them. There seemed to be less of a focus on the supernatural and more of a focus on science, as something more recognizable to modern sensibilities. But, where did this science come from? What body of work were they building on? Where and when did alchemy begin?

Alchemy began as a form of scientific and philosophic practice in at least two distinct locations. It developed in both Egypt and China, independently of one another. In Egypt, alchemy is tied in with the fertility of the Nile River basin, fertility being referred to as Khem. By at least the 4th century BCE, there was a basic practice of alchemy in place, probably related to mummification procedures and connected strongly with ideas of life after death. Much early information on alchemy was lost when the Christians invaded Egypt and burned the library at Alexandria. According to legend, though, the god Thoth was the originator of alchemy in Egypt, and when the Greeks assimilated alchemy into their own practice, Thoth became Hermes-Thoth, who wrote the forty-two books of knowledge, one of which covered alchemy. Hermes symbol was the caduceus, serpent staff, which became a primary symbol of alchemy, and eventually medicine.

Alchemy would not make an appearance in Europe until the 8th century when Muslims finally brought alchemical knowledge with them to Spain. The first European text to mention alchemy appeared in roughly 1050 CE. While Egyptian, Muslim, and European practitioners were certainly interested in the elixir of life, there was a more noticeable focus on creating gold from other substances than was found elsewhere. Gold was perceived to be the perfect metal, with all others being less than perfect. The pursuit of the transmutation of lesser metals into gold was thus also the pursuit of the perfection and transmutation of the human spirit.

One of the most famous of the Islamic alchemists was Jabir ibn Hayyan (Haiyan), who really transformed alchemy through his use of scientific methodology and investigation. Instead of writing in coded words and phrases, Jabir was very straightforward in reporting his activities. In fact, he did not think alchemy was worth pursuing without experimentation. His ultimate goal was the artificial creation of life in the laboratory; he was even willing to accept that it might be possible to create human life in the laboratory.

Alchemy in China was the brainchild of Taoist monks, and as such is wrapped up in Taoist beliefs and practice. The founder of Chinese alchemy is considered to be Wei Po-Yang.

In its earliest practice the Chinese aim was always to discover the elixir of life, not to transmute base metals into gold. Therefore, there was always a closer connection to medicine in China.

When alchemy emerged in China, the word for gold, kim or chim (which referred to the production or creation of gold) was not yet created in the Chinese lexicon. Eventually, the transmutation of other elements into gold was an aim, but it was never the aim in Chinese practice. Additionally, not only were plants and minerals and other substances taken internally, but Chinese alchemy also included exercise techniques that were also meant to help prolong life and manipulate one's life-force. It is probable that the Chinese shared their alchemical practices with interested persons in India (though it is possible that it developed there independently, as well); and as in China, the focus was more often on obtaining the elixir of life than the production of gold.

One of the probable contributions of Chinese alchemists to the world at large is "black powder" or gun powder. This was described as early as the 9th century and used in fireworks within the next 100 years. By the late 13th century, they were using it in cannons. This knowledge first spread to Japan and then farther and farther away, until the Europeans were using gun powder by the 14th century. If this was an alchemical invention, it was likely not the aim, because Chinese alchemy was consistently about medicine, prolonging life, and creating both internal and external balance.

The "Golden Age" of Alchemy

Once Alchemy became known in Spain, it did not take long for information about it to begin working its way through the rest of Europe. Roger Bacon, a 13th century Franciscan Friar, who is considered one of the earliest proponents of the scientific method, is considered the first real European alchemist. (Prior to Bacon, there was some exploration of alchemical theory and ideas, but no real practitioners). He was primarily interested in the elixir of life and some form of ingestible gold which would prolong life. Bacon's writings on alchemy were used by many other practitioners well into the 19th century.

During Bacon's time and for a while after, the church looked at alchemy as a method for exploring theology, and so early European alchemists were clergymen, they being the only ones with enough education to read and decipher the alchemical texts. Unfortunately, Pope John XXII issued an edict banning alchemical counterfeiting, which led to a negative view of alchemical practice within the church. By the 15th century, the English King had banned practice of alchemy without a license.

Once alchemy became more scientific and focused on the transmutation into gold, there was more support for it. This was a period of economic hardship and even many monarchs were hopeful that the claims of alchemy were true. Even the Catholic Church was in favor of alchemical endeavors for this reason. By the 17th and 18th centuries, though, alchemy was decidedly divided into the laboratory practice vs. the philosophical practice, and the laboratory won out. There was no shortage of practitioners in alchemy and related fields. They were involved in all manner of scientific pursuits and most were physicians, professors, metallurgists, or some other profession in addition to being alchemists. They published widely, and often cryptically so as not to reveal too many secrets of the trade. Some authors preferred to publish using pseudonyms, especially adopting the names of famous alchemists and chemists to gain recognition and legitimacy in the field.

Not until the mid-seventeenth century, supposedly with the publication of Robert Boyle's *The Sceptical Chemist*, was there the beginning of a separation between alchemy and chemistry.

And, even then, both were practiced, without distinctions between them, by all manner of scientists, including Isaac Newton, who some consider one of the greatest alchemists of all time. Newton certainly devoted more energy to writing on alchemy than either optics or physics, for which he is best known.

Alchemy, though it largely passed from popularity, continued on. There have been experiments, even into the 20th century, that attempted transmutation, notably using nuclear power and particle acceleration. Pharmacology, while not necessarily admitting to any relationship with alchemy, has as its mission to find the "magic" drugs to help prolong life and heal sickness in much the same way alchemy operated 100s of years ago.

The work done by alchemists forwarded the progress of science on many fronts. The Indian alchemists invented steel and identified metals based on flame color. A famous woman alchemist, Maria the Jewess, from Roman Egypt introduced the use of glass apparatus because it was easier to see what stage the chemicals had reached in any given process. Zosimos, from whom information about Maria the Jewess was revealed, invented a cold still. The modern chemistry laboratory owes a great deal to the many inventions and improvements in lab equipment and processes done for the sake of alchemy.

Alchemists, such as Jabir ibn Haiyan (8th century), extracted anesthetic compounds from herbs, which were used for general anesthesia during operations or difficult procedures. Jabir is also noteworthy for his introduction of a rudimentary elements system which eventually grew, over the centuries, into the table of elements we are familiar with today. Paracelsus, the 15th century physician and alchemist, created laudanum, an opium tincture widely in use until the end of the 19th century. The alchemist Glauber in the 17th century

discovered sodium sulfate, which is also known as "Glauber's salt" and which made him famous. He also was the first to produce concentrated hydrochloric acid and improved the process of manufacturing nitric acid. These are just a few of many alchemists who isolated a variety of natural minerals, elements, and compounds, for a variety of uses. Many of these are crucial elements in modern chemical processes, and these materials could be used in either alchemy or chemistry, if one wants to distinguish between the two.

From today's perspective, the historical origins of spagyrism are unclear. What we do know is that a spagyric medicine already existed in China in the 8th century before Christ; it was based on the alchemical views of the day and in later eras, was also closely connected with Taoism. The situation in ancient India, Persia, Tibet, and naturally in Egypt was similar to that in China. European alchemy and spagyrism was strongly influenced by Egyptian alchemy.

3

Spagyrics

The word spagyric is a composition of the Greek words "spao" = separate and "gyrein" =put together/unite, a part of alchemy which copes with the production of remedies.

Alchemy is a philosophy, which is–for false reasons-reduced to the wrong conception as magic of making gold. Starting from the point of view that the whole creation corresponds to certain laws, the alchemists try to change substances with the aim of imitating natural processes. The word spagyric was firstly used 500 years ago by the medical doctor and philosopher Paracelsus, who regarded health and disease as a misbalance in the harmonious interaction of different principles and who applied his healing methods in order to balance the body again.

Spagyric forms a bridge between classical homeopathy and modern plants science. Although these are two seperate sciences. The energy of the Cosmos is captured in nature by the plants. Spagyric uses these forces of nature to eliminate the blockades, deficits and other pathogenic factors that cause disease.

The use of Spagyric works on the spiritual, mental and physical level. The choice of the element their relationship and degree of dosage determines what happens. Spagyric extracts hit you like a cosmic thunderbolt of healing energy. Spagyrics "opens" the plant and liberates medicine powers not available in the ordinary extract. These medicine powers have nothing to do with the pharmacologically active constituents modern science seeks to standardize.

Both spagyric and ordinary extraction methods macerate (soak) the herb in a menstrum (mixture) of water and grain alcohol between the new and full moon. Water dissolves the water-soluble nutrients; alcohol the alkaloids. The extract is then pressed out, leaving the plant fiber. With ordinary techniques, this fiber or marc is discarded, thus losing the many minerals, trace elements and nutrients, including glycosides, locked up in the cellulose matrix.

The spagyric method cremates the marc in an airtight, oxygen-free kiln at 1500 degrees Fahrenheit for a prolonged period of time (5 or 6 days). This calcination process produces a fine white, mineral rich alkaline ash that is then run (mixed) in a special kind of water, oscillated at a high frequency, pressed out, and allowed to dry into crystals.

Once this running in water process is completed a second time, the crystalline ash is recombined (reunited in the "chymical wedding") back into the original liquid extract, yielding an extremely high potency, fast-acting formula with the full synergy and aroma of the whole living herb and of the etheric cosmic forces that created it.

Why are spagyric extracts infinitely more potent than ordinary ones? Because they release all the nutrients and minerals; because they work with the universal energies of the cosmos; and because they draw upon the spagyric practitioner's mindful intent and inspired heart.

What do you think is the difference between homeopathy and spagyric?

Spagyrics or Plant Alchemy as the medicine has been created by Paracelsus more than 500 years ago, and Homeopathy has been developed by Hahnemann 200 years ago.

Homeopathic mother tincture is made from plant or other natural source. All plants go through the process of maceration for making the liquid homeopathic mother tinctures. After being chopped the fresh plants pieces are placed into a hermetically lockable glass encased grinder together with alcohol. Pure alcohol is used because it is the most effective solvent for extracting the plant's bio-active constituents and delivering them into the bloodstream and across the cell membrane quickly. Many of the plant's constituents are poorly soluble in water, such as resins, essential oils and most alkaloids.

Then the solution or mixture is placed in a dark container or space so that the chemical constituents of the plant are not destroyed. The soaking process can take weeks or even months depending on the substance.

Spaygric essences are made from plants by a unique process, which neutralise their toxic components, but preserves their healing potential. It is concentrated essence, sometimes light colored with the flavor and smells. So the difference between Spagyric and homeopathy is even apparent to our senses, a homoeopathic remedy being hardly differentiable by color, smell or taste from a water-alcohol solution.

Spagyrics means separate and recombine, and can be used to make herbal extracts of great power and energetic force.

Homeopathic mother tinctures are diluted usually in alcohol, then using successive dilutions and succussions of this "mother tincture" potentised dilutions are created with a static or frozen vibrational signature of the original material used, but with none of its physical characteristics.

Plant Alchemy or Spagyrics represents both vital healing energy and active substances which are extracted from medicinal plants, creating powerful mother tinctures that can be further potentized by the circulation process. According to spagyric, every cell has cosmic energies, which make evolution possible. These energies come from the moon, the sun and the stars and need to be gained. Plants consist of 3 parts "body, spirit, soul" – like human beings. The body of a plant is its shape, the etheric substances, which can be gained from plants form the spirit, while smell, taste and color form the soul. These 3 components are separated, purified, concentrated and again unified. This process produced concentrated aromatic solutions that were extracted and separated from the bulk plant matter. After fermentation was completed, the plant material was distilled in a special device, and the remainder dried and burned. The ashes were extracted and purified via distillation, then recombined with the concentrated solution. As a result, the finished spagyric essence contained the mineral constituent parts of the plant. Paracelsus pointed out that the vital energy of an herb is more important than the plant material itself. So spagyric remedies undergo six key steps: separation, purification, distillation, incineration, re-unification and circulation. Through the circulation process the essence gets more ripe and invigorated, or theoretically energized.

Production method consists of very careful distillation, fermentation, purifying, ashing and mixing processes, which are in harmony with certain cosmic cycles.

Fundamentals of Spagyrics

The basic goal in alchemy is called transformation. The basic goal in the alchemy did transformation. The image of the solubilizing lead into gold Alchemists continues to characterize the ideas of this ancient science. The image of making gold from lead alchemists until today characterizes the ideas of this ancient science. The Spagyrics as a medical branch of alchemy is concerned with making from natural raw materials such as plants, minerals and metals, highly active

remedies. The Spagyrics as a branch of medical alchemy deals with natural materials: such as plants, minerals and metals, high-level remedies to make. By certainly pharmacological techniques such as fermentation, distillation and incineration of the starting material to be converted into a particularly healing drug. By certainly pharmacological techniques, color: such as fermentation, distillation and ashing, the starting material in a specially converted healing drugs.

The manufacturers of spagyric medicines rely generally on the traditional writings of Alchemists and Spagyrists of the late Middle Ages and the early modern period. Carl-Friedrich Zimpel (1801-1879), Cesare Mattei (1809-1896), Theodor Krauß -1924) and Alexander von Bernus (1880-1965) were the most significant among them.

4

Principles of Spagyrics

The practice of spagyrics is the application of ancient alchemical working methods to the preparation of tinctures, essences, and other products from medicinal plants. While ordinary tinctures and infusions use only a part of the great curative potential of plants, spagyric methods "open" medicinal plants completely to reveal their more powerful healing properties. Spagyrics includes the Plant Magistery of Paracelsus and the Life Elixir recipe of Andreas Libavius among its historic techniques as well as a wealth of scientific information that demonstrates the greater efficacy of alchemical methods of plant essence extraction. Spagyrics is related to classical alchemical, hermetic and ayurvedic traditions. Spagyric homeopathic remedies act through the neuro-immune-endocrine system and pathways nurturing the reactivity of patients to have the energy to regain health. In traditional Chinese medicine, the elements are wood, fire, earth, metal and water; for the ancient Unani medicine in Arabia, the four humours (akhlaat) are air, earth, fire and water; for Indian ayurvedic medicine, health is the balance of three elemental energies in the universe: air, water and fire. For the ancient Greeks and Romans, these elements were the four bodily fluids or humours. Each corresponded to the four fundamental elements of the world – earth, water, air and fire. In alchemy, Mercury corresponds to water and air, Sulphur corresponds to air and fire, and Salt corresponds to earth and water.

Within the European tradition of phytotherapy there exists two groups of preparations, the spagyric and the homeopathic. The effects of these different preparations differ and somewhat behave as polar opposites to each other. The spagyric expresses the active physical or biochemical components, whereas the homeopathic remedies represent the nonphysical information expressed in the plant. The energy of the cosmos is captured in nature. Spagyrics use these forces of nature to eliminate the blockades, deficits and other pathogenic factors that cause diseases. The use of Spagyrics works on the spiritual, mental and physical level. The choice of the element of their relationship and degree of dosage determines what happens. Spagyric extracts hit like a cosmic thunderbolt of healing energy. Spagyrics "opens" the plant and liberates medicinal powers not available in the ordinary extract. These medicinal powers have nothing to do with the pharmacologically active constituents modern science seeks to standardise. Both spagyric and ordinary extraction methods macerate (soak) the herb in a menstrum (mixture) of water and grain alcohol between the new and full moon. Water dissolves the water soluble nutrients and alcohol the alkaloids. The extract is then pressed out, leaving the plant fibre. With ordinary techniques, this fibre or marc is discarded, thus losing the many minerals, trace elements and nutrients, including glycosides, locked up in the cellulose matrix. The spagyric method cremates the marc in an airtight, oxygen free kiln at 1500 degrees Fahrenheit for a prolonged period of time (five or six days). This calcination process produces a fine white, mineral rich alkaline ash that is then run (mixed) in a special kind of water, oscillated at a high frequency, pressed out, and allowed to dry into crystals. Once this running in water process is completed a second time, the crystalline ash is recombined (re-united in the "chymical wedding") back in to the original liquid extract, yielding an extremely high potency, fast-acting formula with the full synergy and aroma of the whole living herb and of the etheric cosmic forces that created it. Because of the distillation process, Spagyric Essences retain the electrolyte properties of the plants and this is critical to the healing process.

Alchemy has three aspects, Mercury, Sulphur and Salt.

Let's take a look at Mercury. Mercury is considered the Spirit of an object. It is the distinctly aromatic liquid present in all organisms.

The Sulphur is like the Soul of the plant. It's more of the Consciousness.

Salt, according to Robert Allen Bartlett, is the Body of a thing, providing the matrix wherein the Sulphur and Mercury can settle. It is a passive medium, The Virgin Earth, subject to the fixed energies of Water and Earth. Psychic and instinctual forces of the subconscious as well as the conditions affecting the various states of matter influence the Salt. Salt of Aloes is the calcined part obtained from the residue of the cohobation and distillation process of Aloes. German poet and philosopher Goethe writes that detailed knowledge of the chemical composition of a plant alone will not suffice if we do not explore the plant's "spiritual band", i.e., the living secret of its composition and nature.

Spagyric medicine actually pre-dates homeopathy by about two centuries. Homeopathy's father, Samuel Hahnemann, abided by the same basic philosophy but differed in execution. His basic herbal tincture, and that of homeopaths today, is simply the mercurious level of the plant without the minerals and enzymes found in the salt and sulphur levels. Spagyrics is a branch of medicinal alchemy that enhances the healing properties already existing in plants.

Developed by Paracelsus, the magus and alchemist of the early sixteenth century, spagyrics is a holistic therapy that promotes healing at all levels of the human being: body, soul, and spirit. Spagyric essences harness the dynamic life force in plants that triggers recovery from the energetic imbalance of illness. The harmonising and balancing qualities of spagyric essences differ from other plant remedies and aromatherapy oils because they not only include the plant's energetic information but also incorporate the salt of the plant, from which all toxic matter has been purged. The preparation of this alchemical medicine makes it possible to capture the full therapeutic spectrum of plants, including the cosmic energies they have absorbed. These essences work holistically to heal the mind, body, and spirit with the energetic qualities of the plant or the electrolytes. The original rationale behind these special herbal tinctures seems to have been that an extract using alcohol could not be expected to contain all the medicinal properties from a living plant, and so the ash or mineral component (as a result of the calcination process) of the calcined plant was prepared separately and then added back to "augment" (increase) the alcoholic tincture. Herbal tinctures are typically alcoholic extracts of a plant or plants, although some varieties are made with vinegar, glycerol, ether, or some other material. Compared to homeopathic or herbal, spagyric tinctures are arguably more versatile in their use because they are always nontoxic and gentle. Spagyric tinctures are easy to use internally and externally as complementary remedies. These remedies stimulate with their spagyric phytocomponents, which provide an extra energy boost and regulate via the homeopathic properties of individual plant constituents. This powerful combination creates "super-charged" remedies that invigorate the body's vital energy, act as immune system catalysts and promote more efficient cellular activity to help infected or weakened organ tissues resume normal function.

Plant alchemy or Spagyrism represents a form of medicine in which both vital healing energy and active substances are extracted from medicinal plants, creating powerful tinctures that can be further potentised through circulation.

Od Force is the cosmic life force that animates and circulates throughout creation; natural electromagnetic energy of the infinite universe consisting of positive, negative and neutral charges which build and sustain the human body and all other matter. Everyone is surrounded by an electromagnetic field, and this field is called an aura. The aura has been depicted throughout history in literature and paintings. Angel pictures show it as a halo; pictures of Gods often depict a light around his head. Auras are not unique to angels and religious leaders, however; a field of energy surrounds us all. This is called Prana in Ayurveda, meaning primary energy. It is sometimes translated as breath or vital force, though it is more than these. This life force energy is represented as qi (chi) in traditional Chinese medicine. The homeopathic notion of the Vital Force is a spirit-like essence that animates a living organism. In homeopathy, disease is considered to originate as a disruption of the vital force. Symptoms produced are thought to reflect the nature of the disruption. It is an innate intelligence that is not entirely physical or spiritual. As there is order to the universe based on energy, so must our internal order or Vital Force energy be in balance. When it is not, disease results and symptoms develop. Symptoms of disease are an outer expression of our inner disrupted Vital Force. These symptoms are helpful clues to which areas of our body need attention. The body has the ability to heal itself and this knowledge is within all of our cells or neuro-immuno-endocrine system as physiologists say.

Most traditional healing practices posited that disease was the result of some imbalance in the vital energies which distinguish living from non-living matter.

Od force is the laws of energy that govern our life, so what is it that makes life? What is the difference between a dead body and a living person? Is it the Od Force an active principle forming part of any living thing. The life energy is so strong that scientists have theorized that disease within the physical body actually occurs at the cellular and bimolecular levels. In this scenario, healing extends from the bimolecular level to the cellular and finally, to the anatomical.

This is because the bimolecular properties of the physical body are based on vibration. The vibration of the life-force, which we receive through our five senses, possess electromagnetic properties. Mitogenic energy (mitosis) is generated in the form of electromagnetic energy, which creates the energy of light (ethereal fluid) that surrounds each cell.

German scientist Dr. Wilhelm Reich researched the nature of this energy in the 1940's and unraveled many of its secrets. He came to realise the sensitive living nature of this cosmic life energy as the essence of creation, the force that holds it all together, from the energy of our souls to the invisible force that keeps planets in their orbits. It is this energy that creates our feelings and our moods. In addition the weather is created by the constant cyclical movements of this energy.

The science of bio magnetism refers to the measurement of magnetic fields produced by living organisms. These tiny magnetic fields are produced by naturally occurring electric currents resulting from muscle contraction, or signal transmission in the nervous system, or by the magnetization of biological tissue.

Every substance and organism radiates and absorbs energy via a unique wave field, which then exhibits certain geometrical frequency and radiation characteristics.

There is a measurable, extended force field that exists around all forms of matter, whether animate or inanimate. Dr. Mitchell May found that life force energy manifested as specific patterns and structures. Those plants with the brightest, most intricate and most well-balanced energy, such as particular herbs, enzymes, algae, mushrooms and sprouts, were the same botanicals used by traditional healers. Their unusually radiant and harmonic patterns seemed to be valuable reservoirs of pure life force energy. Kirlian photography shows a beautiful, circle-shaped vibratory image that appears in certain plants when they are at their peak of flowering. Plants harvested too early or too late won't reveal this type of harmonic image. Thus when these healing herbs are expertly grown, harvested, prepared and blended together, they transfer their inherent patterns into our energetic fields and greatly enhance our health and well-being.

The potency and quality of a natural herbal product thus depends upon harvesting its ingredients at the optimal time. German spagyrist Baron Alexander Von Bernus, wrote on this subject, in his fascination book: Alchemy and Medicine, that the current knowledge of the plants called an organica (containing a lot of mineral salts) that act as remineralizer producing an exchange of element in human body, should have allowed a deep study of the prime importance of the salts that constitute the mineral substance of vegetal.

Energy medicine is a domain in CAM that deals with energy fields of two types: Veritable, and Putative, the veritable energies employ mechanical vibrations (such as sound) and electromagnetic forces, including visible light, magnetism, monochromatic radiation and rays from other parts of the electromagnetic spectrum.

They involve the use of specific, measurable wavelengths and frequencies to treat patients.

Putative energy fields have defied measurement to date by reproducible methods. Therapies involving putative energy fields are based on the concept that human beings are infused with a subtle form of energy. This vital energy or life force is known under different names in different cultures, such as qi in traditional Chinese medicine, the vital energy or life force proposed to regulate a person's spiritual, emotional, mental, and physical health and to be influenced by the opposing forces of yin and yang, in traditional Chinese medicine. A whole medical system that originated in China. It is based on the concept that disease results from disruption in the flow of qi and imbalance in the forces of yin and yang. Practices such as herbs, meditation, massage, and acupuncture seek to aid healing by restoring the yin-yang balance and the flow of qi (TCM), ki in the Japanese Kampo system, doshas in Ayurvedic medicine. A whole medical system that originated in India. It aims to integrate the body, mind, and spirit to prevent and treat disease.

Therapies used include herbs, massage, and yoga, and elsewhere as prana, etheric energy, fohat, orgone, odic force and homeopathic resonance. Vital energy is believed to flow throughout the material human body, but it has not been unequivocally measured by means of conventional instrumentation. Nonetheless, therapists claim that they can work with this subtle energy, see it with their own eyes, and use it to effect changes in the physical body and influence health.

Practitioners of energy medicine believe that illness results from disturbances of these subtle energies. An energy field that is proposed to surround and flow throughout the human body and play a role in health. Acupuncture, Reiki and qi gong are examples of therapies that involve bio electricity.

Spagyric homeopathy is one approach with implications for energy medicine. Spagyric homeopathy is often termed as 'Electro-Alchemy' to "make homeopathic remedies and combination homeopathic remedies in low potency". The principle underlying remedy making is based on the understanding that all physical substances have a unique energy pattern. This also applies to Spagyric Homeopathic remedies produced pharmaceutically. Practitioners believe that their remedies mobilize the body's vital force to orchestrate coordinated healing responses throughout the organism. The body translates the information on the vital force into local physical changes that lead to recovery from acute and chronic diseases. Practitioners use their assessment of the deficits in vital force to guide dose (potency) selection and treatment pace, and to judge the likely clinical course and prognosis.

Alchemists conceive the universe as being Divine and the manifestation of the one God. Nature and its laws are the very outer expression of the Godhead. In the words of the Kybalion, 'The All is Mind, the Universe is mental'. In order to obtain a clear concept of what the 3 principles of Salt, Sulphur and Mercury mean in the preparation of Spagyric Medicine, remember that the mercury principle is similar to the extraction medium in the case of dry plant material as the Sulphur is to the extracted phytochemicals. The salt principle is extracted from the ashes of the plant.

All manifestation exists by virtue of dual forces. Perception and conception can only exist where an object is relative to, and in contrast with another. Some specific examples are:

'As above, so below'. This is a great law having many applications. It is the law of correspondence of the planes, indicating that whatever exists and is created in the inner worlds (as well as celestial influences) is reflected simultaneously in the outer physical reality. Once this is accepted as a living law, the activity occurring on the inner psychic planes can be accurately ascertained by observation of the events, objects and relationships that come into outer life. True awareness of this law obliges us to take responsibility for every aspect of our lives. If an outer circumstance is felt to be inharmonious, then it can be changed effectively by inner plane work. 'As below, so above' indicates that our outer actions have a corresponding effect on the inner planes (this leads to so-called *Karma*). Laboratory work, i.e., manipulation and regeneration of physical substances and elements, etc., leads to the transmutation of the corresponding psychic archetypes. Jung termed the Alchemist's concerns with physical matter, 'projections of the unconscious' onto that matter, which is valid, but only halfway there.

Everything in the universe consists of two polar opposites; everything has an opposite pole to itself, where the poles differ only in degree. A simple illustration is heat and cold, which are different degrees of the same thing temperature. Where does heat begin and cold end? What we see as hot and cold depends on the situation, so we may conclude that it is a matter of relativity. Manifestations of heat and cold, light and darkness, love and hate, fear and courage, good and evil are 'merely a form, variety and rate of vibration', as it is put in The Kybalion. It is possible to effect a change of one pole to another within this 'form, variety or rate of vibration'. It is the detested weakness in ourselves, that once transmuted become our very strengths, to push us on toward the One.

All creation, generation and regeneration is not possible without the male/female principles interacting. Every female contains a male principle, and every male, the female.

The Trinity of Alchemy

Of primary concern to the Alchemist are the three essentials, or great trinity which comprise all manifestation. In alchemical literature they are the much confused Mercury, Sulphur, Salt, and are often referred to as the Three-in-One.

a. Mercury (Spirit) Mercury, to an Alchemist is the most important concept and physical essence. It is not to be confused with ordinary metallic mercury, and is known under a variety of names, such as Water of Life, Prima Material, Water of the Wise, Philosophical Mercury, Seed, Heavenly Water and Azoth. In simple terms Mercury is, as everything is polar in nature.

The water, alcohol and alkahest serve as vehicles, in their respective kingdoms, of the life-force, thus when the alchemist works with these substances, he is working with living entities.

Alkahest is described as an inflammable, clear, very volatile liquid which is contained wholly within the mineral. In the Collectanae Chemica (Anon), mercury is spoken of thus:

'All true philosophers agree that the first Matter of metals is a moist vapour raised by the action of the central fire in the bowels of the earth, which, circulating through its pores meets with the crude air, and is coagulated by it into an unctuous water adhering to the earth which serves it for a receptacle, where it is joined to a sulphur more or less pure and a salt more or less fixing, which it attracts from the air, and, receiving a certain degree of concoction from the central and solar heat is formed into stones and rocks, mineral and metals.

Hence it appears that the first Matter of metals is one thing and not many, homogenous, but altered by the diversity of places and sulphurs with which it is combined.'

Mercury is thus the archetypal idea of all entity, just as the idea of flower exists above and before the manifest flower (the seed contains the fruit) and Adam exists above and before terrestrial man. In terms of gender, the Mercury is of feminine polarity (but contains within it certain masculine characteristics), symbolised by the moon.

b. Sulphur (Soul) Again, it must be understood that the sulphur referred to here is not common one.

It is the role of Sulphur to coagulate; and to concentrate the life-force in one physical location. The organisational aspect of Sulphur maintains the human organism with its different organs as one cohesive unit. Macro-cosmically solar gravitational attraction sustains the orbits of the planets which maintains the harmony and rhythm of the solar system unit. In the Collectanae Chemica 'these three kingdoms do not indeed differ in their virtue nor the three sulphurs, as every sulphur has the power to coagulate its own Mercury; and every Mercury has a power of being coagulated by its own proper sulphur, and by none other which is a stranger to it.'

Sulphur has the masculine polarity attributed to it, symbolised by the sun.

c. Salt (Body) Salt is the substance that exoteric science deals with exclusively, but it is not common table salt. It is the familiar salts of the mineral kingdom as well as the mineral ash of the plant and animal kingdoms. The non-physical polarity is the subtle vehicle, in all three kingdoms.

If the human organism did not possess a fascinatingly great self-healing capability, all of our therapeutic efforts would be for nothing. Even with diseases which as far as anyone can judge are certain to be fatal, spontaneous healing sometimes occurs. The capability of the organism for regeneration and self-healing must not be underestimated. We must investigate the basic causes of these self-healing processes; for here is where the therapy must exert its effect. Basically, only the human organism can heal itself; as therapists, supporting these self-healing processes is our primary function.

To provide support for self-healing in the holistic sense, it is essential to search for the underlying causes of the disease.

Naturally, there are many reasons why diseases develop. Paracelsus (Theophrast von Hohenheim) stressed-more than half a millennium ago-five factors that cause diseases to develop. He called these disease causes entien. To my knowledge, the paracelsian entien correspond to the following factors:

1. Physical, climatic, geographical influences
2. Toxic influences
3. Constitution and disposition (genetics)
4. Psychosomatic causes
5. Superordinate to these first 4 factors is the quintessence, Paracelsus's ens dei, now also commonly referred to with the concept of *karma*.

In addition,, there were 4 levels, i.e., Earth, Water, Fire and Spirit, which are very important for diagnosis and treatment in Spagyrism.

Spagyrism can be described as a distinct branch of holistic because diagnosis and therapy start from the concept of a unified whole consisting of body, life, soul and spirit, what lies behind these concepts is regarded as reality. Above all in the early pre-pharmacological era in which spagyrism came into being, human beings regarded themselves as such quadripartite beings. That was possible because mankind lived in an entirely different state of consciousness than is true today.

Basically, we must realize that what we perceive of the world can only be a segment of reality and that we modify our perception of this segment in ways corresponding to our consciousness.

Spirit and soul have been declared as non-existent in the modern natural sciences because the ability to perceive them has been lost; materialism is narrowing our field of vision more and more. This has consequences in many fields-in medicine and drug research as well. The logical consequence of the materialistic and mechanistic way of thinking is that medicaments are defined exclusively in material, that is, chemical terms.

The Starting Substances

Spagyrism is a holistic medicine because in producing its medicaments, only natural substances are used.

For the production of spagyric preparations, only natural substances are used; here, great attention is given to origin and quality. Substances which do not come from nature sources have no relevance to human evolution. In a certain sense, they can be referred to as dead materials which are unable to engage in fruitful communication with actual life processes.

In detail, the natural substances used are the following: Fresh plants, wax, gum, mucilage, tannins, resins, etc., Naturally occurring minerals and rocks, Native metals, Compounds produced from natural substances in spagyric laboratories, Animals and their substances.

All materials employed should have as natural an origin as possible: from gathering in the wild or from biological cultivation. Spagyrism justifies the use of the drugs which are normally intended for phytotherapeutic application.

Nowadays, it is best to produce the medicinal plants using spagyric-biological cultivation. For some medicinal herbs, gathering in the wild is no longer acceptable because it fosters the eradication of the plants or at least represents a major intervention in the balance of nature.

For the spagyric-biological cultivation of medicinal herbs, nature should always be followed as the model.

If possible, medicinal plants that are used for cultivation should have a wide variety is desired here. Therefore, the plants should not be reproduced from root division or using cuttings. Seeds should always be used for reproduction.

It is very good to use medicinal plant seeds of the same type but from different regions for growing young plants.

It is equally important to harvest certain species only every 2nd or 3rd year. The plants should be allowed to form seeds that germinate to form new plants.

Throughout organic farming is advised, chemical fertilizers, insecticides, herbicides, and fungicides should not be used (insist on biological cultivation or gathering from the wild). Since, spagyric preparations are based on the plant vitality the time of collection of medicinal herbs are calculated not only on their flowering season, but to mystic astrological calculations.

It must be particularly taken into account that the medicinal plants should be harvested in the developmental stage that is ideal for efficacy. This assumes special knowledge of the natural rhythms.

By means of spagyric medicinal plant cultivation, areas can be created which represent a popular living area for many endangered animals, particularly many insects and birds. It creates areas which are free from toxic substances and not intensively cultivated.

5
The Quest for the Quintessence

"the history of spagyrical philosophy begins with Albertus Magnus, Baymund Lully and Roger Bacon, of the thirteenth century, but reached its highest development under Paracelsus."

The characteristics of esoteric science are said to be: "The principle of analogy and its consequences; the relation of the forces and the laws of the macrocosm to those of the microcosm; logical investigation both experimental and speculative; the reciprocity of cause and effect determining the oscillations of blind chance." Only students of these principles are able to apply the mysterious remedies of the new therapeutics so as fully to secure miraculous efficiency.

An important factor in alchemical philosophy is the influence of the sun, moon and planets on diseases; the moon especially excites dreams, insomnia, somnambulism, and governs the periodicity of fevers. But the most potent of all celestial influences is the 'odic-magnetic virtue of the stars.'

A notable feature, overlooked by official medicine, but rescued from oblivion by the promoters of Electro-Homeopathy, is the peculiar way in which 'odic force' is distributed in the human body; it flows along three principal axes, head to feet, left side to right side and back to chest; this polarized fluid is assimilated by the five vegetable electricities, which explains their efficiency.

Physicians who appreciate the importance of the 'three axes of odic-magnetic polarity 'place their patients in bed on their right sides (—), with their heads (—) to the north (+) and their faces (+) to the wall.

The chemical philosophy of this school has the merit of simplicity; the unity of matter and the four ancient elements are the basic principles. Fire is hydrogen; Air is oxygen; Water is nitrogen, and Earth is carbon; the alchemical salts, sulphur and mercury are respectively the principles of solidity, volatility and liquidity. The Alkahest, or universal solvent, of spagyrical philosophy is acetone; the spiritus philosophorum is not merely a liquid of superior medicinal potency, it is the "true spirit of the knowledge of control over Nature's forces, which results from unions with and absorption by the Divine Being."

The position of modern alchemists with reference to the transmutation of metals is entirely favorable to the ancient doctrine. "Modern science," writes one, "regards the creation of gold as a superstitious fable, the product of medieval imaginations, but transmutation is an undeniable fact; a family beloved by the author preserves as a relic an ingot of gold, which an ancestor, initiated in the secrets of Hermetism, had manufactured by a formula now intelligible only to adepts." L 1 Hyperchimie, the organ of alchemists in France, has added Electro-Homoeopathy to the subjects it advocates, and contains an enthusiastic review of the latest treatise on this medical practice; the review concludes with the remark that: "Occult therapeutics is destined to become the system of the future, as it has been that of the past, for it demonstrates with invincible logic the admirable unity of the sacred sciences."

(Iatro-Chemistry in 1897, Bolton, H. Carrington Science, Volume 7, March 25, 1898).

The Great Work of alchemy lies chiefly in the quest for a mysterious substance known as the Quintessence (from the Medieval Latin quinta essentia or "fifth essence"). This substance is believed to possess many seemingly miraculous properties, being capable of granting longevity to the alchemist, transforming base metals to gold, and curing all diseases. Alchemists believe that the seed of this Quintessence may be found in all matter, but that it is more easily extracted from certain base substances. These substances, reduced to a primal form called "hyle" or the First Matter, are then subjected to gentle heating until the Stone emerges from this chaotic mass.

The Emerald Tablet of Hermes, a short text composed of a number of enigmatic verses ascribed to the God Hermes, is said to form the essential core of alchemical philosophy. Through it we learn that the process of alchemy is essentially transformational. Furthermore, it states that there is a correspondence between that which is Above and that which is Below, which can be understood through a study of astrology and the processes of nature, reflected in both the macrocosmic world and in the microcosm of the alchemist. The alchemist always works in partnership with Nature, to accelerate these processes which otherwise would take millennia to reach fruition, and draw those natural forces into the experiment through the principle of correspondence.

In laboratory alchemy, the experiments of transformation occur simultaneously in both the material being manipulated and in the alchemist's soul.

The next section uses the alchemical work in the Plant kingdom to illustrate the fundamental principles of the Art.

Trees have an interesting role in the world of spirituality. Many people may instantly think about the practice of decorating a Christmas tree, but that is just one example. Trees have been held sacred in many cultures both ancient and modern. Both beautiful and symbolic, trees are very powerful and can influence our spiritual lives.

Taoist Masters observed that trees are tremendously powerful plants. Not only can they absorb carbon dioxide and transform it into oxygen, but they can also absorb negative forces and transform them into good energy. Trees strongly root with the Earth, and the more rooted the tree, the higher it can extend to Heaven. Trees stand very still, absorbing the Earth's Energy and the Universal Force from the Heavens.

Trees and all plants have the ability to absorb the light of the energies and transform it into food; in fact, they depend on light for most of their nourishment, while water and earth minerals make up about 30% of their nutritional intake. Trees are able to live very long lives.

Trees are the largest and most spiritually advanced plants on earth. They are constantly in meditation, and subtle energy is their natural language. As your understanding of this language grows, you can begin to ascertain stomatal control, phototropism, photomorphogenic growth and environmental signaling.

Throughout history human beings have used all parts of the tree for healing and medicine. The best trees for healing are big trees, especially pines. Pine trees radiate Qi, nourish blood, strengthen nervous systems, and contribute to long lives. They also nurture souls and spirits.

Among the most powerful are trees growing near running water. Some trees feel warmer or hotter than others; some feel cooler or colder than others.

6

Plant Alchemy

Spagyrics is a way of separating and preserving the hidden qualities (signatures) of plants and minerals in elixirs, tinctures, and powders. The results are subtle yet powerful medicines free of the impurities normally associated with their gross material forms.

We have chosen to describe the processes of creating the vegetable Stone as shown by Junius, as these are well documented (and are the only processes with which I am familiar!). They mirror and mimic the same processes used in mineral alchemy, so that once the vegetable Stone has been made, the alchemist is ready to tackle the Great Work.

The following table shows a brief description of the Three Principles as they are used in alchemical work. They are universal in scope and preformative in nature. The properties of these Principles are listed as they are generally understood by modern alchemists such as Junius, Albertus and Dubuis.

Sulfur

Sulfur is the Principle which determines the unique identity of the Matter. It is considered to be the "soul", that which carries the consciousness. It possesses the quality of Heat and is considered to be the Masculine principle.

Salt

Salt is the Principle which provides structure, the ability to distinguish the particular constituents of the Matter. Alchemists sometimes call this the "Secret Fire", because although Salt appears to be static, it conceals a volatile, dynamic essence which, when released, causes the Three Principles to reunite in the creation of the Stone.

Mercury

Mercury is the Principle which connects everything, and which is receptive to the dynamic activity of Sulfur. It is considered to be anonymous, unlike the Sulfur, and is said to be the "same everywhere", ubiquitous and undifferentiated. It has the property of Cold and is the Feminine principle in alchemy.

It is through the skillful separation and recombination of the Principles that the alchemist seeks to recreate the First Matter out of which the Stone may flower.

The Plant Stone

This is a brief overview of the creation of the Plant Stone as described by Mark Stavish, analyzed from the viewpoint of each of the Principles, using colored markup to highlight the Principle being manipulated.

Separating the Sulfur

The Sulfur of the plant is carried in its essential oils, which are highly volatile. Therefore, these oils are separated from the plant using steam distillation and kept aside. They will be rejoined to the other separated Principles later. This process also "opens up" the Sulfur, expanding it both physically and energetically in order that latent properties may have space to become manifest.

Fermenting the Mass

The remainder of the plant, reduced to a watery mass by distillation, is now placed in a fermenting vessel in a warm, dark place. The goal here is to cause the plant Mercury, carried in the form of alcohol, to arise in the mass.

Unless a very great quantity of plant material is present, though, there will be very little plant sugar to feed the yeast that produces alcohol. Therefore, the alchemist will add raw sugar, as well as a quantity of brewer's yeast. This is allowed because, as stated above, the Mercury Principle is the "same everywhere", and the sugar that is transformed into alcohol bears the seed of this Principle.

Separating the Salts

Once the fermentation is complete (the yeast stops bubbling), the solids are separated by filtration and set aside to dry. These will later yield mineral salts which carry the Salt Principle.

Distilling the Mercury

The watery "soup" left behind by separation is then distilled, gently, extracting the alcohol. The alchemists say that the plant Mercury has been "determined" by the process of fermentation, meaning that its original anonymity (remember, Mercury is anonymous and the "same everywhere") is replaced with specificity.

The distillation process also "opens up" the Mercury; during this process, the intent of the alchemist may be more easily impressed upon the determined Mercury.

Separating the Fixed Sulfur

The remaining "soup" is then evaporated until it forms a viscous liquid. This is then subjected to greater heat, resulting in a blackened, solid mass (note the parallel with the black phase or "Nigredo" mentioned earlier). Further heating ("calcination") causes it to gradually whiten. This is further divided into water soluble salts, called the "fixed Sulfur", and insoluble salts, the caput mortuum or dead head of these salts.

Reducing the Salts

Next, the solids in the plant mass are roasted, calcined, and separated into soluble salts (the vegetable Salt) and insoluble caput mortuum. Typically, the insoluble salts are discarded.

Coagula: Confecting the Stone

Finally, the soluble salts are mixed together, and the essential oils and alcohol gently added to them ("imbibing") until the salts can take up no more of the liquids. The resulting clay like Matter is then placed in the crucible and heated gently until it turns bright red, signaling the creation of the Stone. This process is very similar to the one described in the "Collectanea", and requires similar skills and sensitivity.

Inner Processes

Throughout the work, the alchemist must dwell on the materials and processes, until she is truly experiencing this transformation from plant to Stone. Without this inner involvement, the process will fail. Though in the above experiment, the "coagula" phase seems short, it is the most challenging and delicate, requiring great sensitivity of the alchemist to produce the Philosopher's Stone.

7
Energetic Spagyrics

According to Spagyrics, vital energy can be separated into 7 main vibratory frequencies. These 7 frequencies, or rays, or bio-energies or vital energies are all symbolically linked to a colour, a planet, thus the importance of astrology in Spagyric medicine.

These 7 vital energies correspond to states of consciousness and each living thing is linked to one or another-or to several of these energies according to their own vibratory state.

In the human body, these 7 vital energies govern the organs, but also the physiological and and psychological functions.

In nature, each of these 7 frequencies are in vibratory affinity with certain minerals and certain plants.

Spagyrics help to understand the correspondences between plants and the vital energies to which they are linked. When a disequilibrium happens in the circulation of vital energy, by identifying the weakened energy thanks to an energetic evaluation, Spagyrics work by reinforcing the weakened energy by an appropriate energetic boost. Spagyric remedies, which preserve and dynamize the vital essence of plants, are specially made to provide this energetic boost and re-establish the circulation of vital energy.

The 7 vital energies are the following:

Depleting energy:

Depleting energy preside in relations with the environment. It is linked to communication, evolution, adaptation to changes and new things introduced into the environment.

Depleting energy govern the ability to adapt, as well as mental and physical flexibility. At an organic level, depleting energy is linked to the neurosensorial system and to the respiratory system.

Purifying energy:

Purifying energy is linked to regeneration in relation with the maternal archetype, the subconscious world and the oneiric.

At an organic level, purifying energy is linked to the lymphatic system, to the gonads, to the bone marrows, to the digestive tube and to organic liquids.

Harmonizing energy:

Harmonizing energy is an energy that structures and divides up the energetic flow in an organism. It is in relation with power, justice and authority.

At an organic level, harmonizing energy is linked to connective tissues, to muscular tissues and to the liver.

Calming energy:

Calming energy is represented by the feminine archetype. It is in relation with sensibility, receptivity and beauty.

Calming energy governs anti-inflammatory reactions, and in a more general manner, shape physiological and psychological reactions in response to external aggressions.

At an organic level, calming energy is linked to the urinary system, to the vein system, to the mucous membranes, and to the female sexual organs.

Dynamizing energy:

Dynamizing energy is linked to the masculine archetype. It is in relation with willpower, force, the desire to fight, conquest and competition. Dynamizing energy governs defense reactions in response to external aggressions.

At an organic level, dynamizing energy is linked to the gallbladder, to the immune system, to the artery system and to the male sexual organs.

Securing energy:

Securing energy is an energy that helps to anchor oneself to reality, in relation with the paternal archetype, rationality and practical sense.

At an organic level, it corresponds with the colon, the bones, the tendons, and the appendages.

Illuminating energy:

Illuminating energy is in relation with personal development, with the expression of personality, with equilibrium and integration of all other forms of vital energy.

At an organic level, illuminating energy is linked to the heart and the eyes.

In the Indian Ayurveda medicine, we can still find alchemical views and preparation processes today, and particularly in the Southern Indian Siddha medicine as well. Viewed from the spagyric point of view, particularly the botanical preparation processes of contemporary Ayurveda medicine are unfortunately carried out on a qualitatively very low level.

The intellectual origin of spagyrism lies in alchemy. Alchemy is based on ancient wisdom concerning the earth, cosmos, and man, which is also referred to as the science of life in the material universe. One should not be deterred by the term, alchemy. With it is not meant the distorted image of a degenerated alchemy that has shaped our ideas from the Middle Ages down to the present century. In reality, alchemy is a magnificent philosophical and (in the truest sense of the word) scientific edifice that many peoples have helped to erect.

The science of life in the material universe was given different names in different cultures and ages. In Europe it is referred to as alchemy (Alchymie).

To the extent that alchemical work dealt practically with prophylaxis, diagnosis, the production of medicaments, and treatment, one talked of spagyrism.

Accordingly, spagyrism is the practical application of alchemy in medical treatment.

The word, spagyrism, that we use today probably first came into existence in the Middle Ages. It is derived from the Greek and means something like separate or divide and unite or bind. This separation and uniting is of significance to spagyrism on all levels. Indeed it is the significance of life processes for example expiration and inspiration.

One of the most famous spagyrists was Theophrast von Hohenheim, called Paracelsus. However, during this period and later, there were many other spagyrists who are no longer familiar today because their work did not come to public attention.

Substance, Information, Power

To understand spagyrism, it is appropriate to distinguish between three levels: these are:

1. The material or molecular level
2. The information level
3. The powers level

Please note that these levels cannot actually be viewed as being completely separate from one another. However, to understand their relationship to one another, it is simpler to discuss them one by one.

1. The Substance Level

Here, we must consider the purely physical effect of chemically defined medicaments. This is the level with which modern pharmacology is concerned. In practical drug research, the conscious concentration on this level alone leads to the active chemico-synthetic agents and also to pure plant substances which, like the other chemical compounds, are employed above all for substitution and suppression. As a rule, they exert a clear pharmacological effect, which says nothing however about whether they also possess a therapeutic efficacy.

In human beings, certain chemical substances produce an narcotized state similar to sleep by means of blocking the production or transmission of messenger substances: suppression. For this reason, traditional medicine uses such substances with sleep disturbances. Apart from the well-known side effects (e.g. liver damage, disturbance of the rapid eye movement sleep phase, hangover, dependence, etc.), an acquired tolerance develops relatively quickly, which requires increasing the dose. What is interesting, however, is that after discontinuance of the drug, the sleep disturbances are as a rule considerably more severe than before the therapy. In reality, the medicament employed had no curative influence on the disorder and it was therefore not therapeutically effective; the sleep disturbances were only masked.

2. The Information Level

Whereas the production of chemically defined medicaments takes only the substance level into account, homeopathy concentrates above all on the information level.

According to homeopathic ideas, a vehicle substance (ethanol/water, lactose, or something similar) is impregnated with the structure of a certain primary substance. This impregnated primary substance information is intended to stimulate a reaction in the organism by which the healing process is initiated.

Our consciousness, emotions and apprehension influence our neuro-immuno-endocrine system. In several traditional medicines, incl. Ayurveda, Homeopathy and Acupuncture disease is considered to originate as a disruption of the life force or the core information matrix. If there is a disorder in the information level, diseases will occur. In human body brain is the core information matrix. Everything in our universe is inter-connected by information-subtle-energy wave fields.

Any imbalance of the life force comes from well within our own consciousness. Health could be obtained by removing the distracted information level or consciousness.

The psychological phenomena consists of the totality of the mind, thought, connection and spiritual emotions. The changes and events in these worlds are projected onto our somatic body (Sigmund Freud, Carl Gustav Jung).

Spagyric medicines when applied therapeutically transmit information of the trace elements and are able to penetrate and correct the energy level in the living organisms and influence at the deepest informational state, respectively the DNAs and RNAs, the higher states of emotional and physical health, thus, influence limbic activity, then hypothalamus and pituitary gland, and finally the sexual organs and adrenal glands. Based on the principle of quantum physics, subtle energy information of spagyric essences influence and harmonize the elemental information levels of the consciousness, emotions, behavior, thoughts, connections, soul and spirit, from DNA to cells, it harmonize our energy fields. This is possible on the information level or better, on the false information level.

3. The Powers Level

Now we come to the level of the powers. For spagyrism, the powers level is of paramount importance, and by means of the spagyric production methods, specific healing powers are developed from natural substances.

We must assume that something like a primordial power, an elemental force, exists. This primordial and universal life energy is present in the cosmos, in the atmosphere, in water, in every mineral, every plant, every animal, and every human being. However, it is not always present in the same form. Every natural substance and naturally every organism corresponds to a highly specific modification of this originally universal vital energy. Such a vital force was known to many cultures and peoples.

Chi was influenced with the help of acupuncture. In Japan, this energy was called *Ki*, the Indians referred to *Prana*, Baron von Reichenbach called it *Od*, and Wilhelm Reich, *Orgon*. In alchemy (Alchymie) we call it *Chy*. Whether or not all of these terms refer to exactly the same thing has not yet been investigated. However, these concepts at least included the different revelations or effects of this elemental force. The presence of specific vital powers or vital energies is what also differentiates natural substances from synthetic substances. The specific healing power of a natural substances is of course quite different than that of a petrochemical/synthetic or similar substance, if one indeed can speak of the healing power of such dead substances.

The energy which represents to a certain extent the basic component of this universal vital force can be termed electricity. This term was used accordingly by spagyrists like Krauß, Mattei, and Glückselig around the turn of the century. This force or better, these healing powers are important for therapeutic regeneration. They are also effective when the vital capability to respond to information is lacking.

With the aid of spagyric processes, natural metallic, mineral, and botanical substances are used to develop medicaments with indication-specific healing powers whose site of action lies in the realm of the living processes.

A constitution is not a disease. It is the idiosyncratic genetic character modified by the sum total of the spiritual, mental, and physical impregnations. In terms of prophylaxis, the spagyric preparations are administered for strengthening the constitution.

Disposition refers to the individual tolerance against illness-producing stimuli. The weakest organ is the first to react pathologically to strong stimuli. By the application of spagyric preparations, the individual tolerance can be increased.

The term, diathesis, refers to the inability to compensate for even weak stimuli. Certain organs or organ systems represent the weakest link in the chain and break when placed even under only mild stress. By means of the appropriate ways of living and therapy, diatheses can be lastingly compensated for.

The so-called weaknesses are connected with these factors. Weaknesses always represent a lack of vital energy. This can be a general deficit or a deficit located only in the region of an organ or organ system.

In young people and with a reasonable life-style, no disease develops. However, after decades or in crisis situations, a true disease can develop. In these patients, there is a tendency to migraines, neuroses, gastric and cardiac diseases, etc. Prophylactically as well as therapeutically, it is important to treat the causes, which lie in the sensitive weakness of the neuro-immuno-endocrine system.

By means of spagyric preparations which are aimed at effecting the central nervous system (CNS), an organ-specifically modified healing power can be supplied to the CNS. This healing and strengthening effect proves indeed to be therapeutically efficacious in practice, for sleep disturbances as well, within the context of holistic therapy (i.e. taking account of differing causes). In spagyric therapy, first priority is given to strengthening the weak points by supplying specific healing powers for so long that they are again in a position to carry out their functions on their own.

In practice, spagyric preparations are most appropriate for holistic healing; for they exert effects on all three levels because due to the specific steps in the preparation process, the material substance level, information level, and powers level are preserved and in part strengthened. Since the effect of these remedies are on the three levels of healing, they can also be used to therapeutically induce organisms which have a lack of the vital ability to react to energy field.

Spagyric medicines are energy accumulators which contain an indication-specifically modified healing power. They are related to the chemically defined medicines by their material basis, and to the homeopathic remedies by the intensive impregnation with information concerning the primary substance. But they only become genuine spagyric remedies by means of the development of specific healing powers.

In comparison to the treatment with chemically defined medicaments, a physiological process, for example, is not simulated, but rather regenerated with spagyric medicine.

In contrast to classic homoeopathic treatment, no vital energy for responding to the healing stimulus is required from the organism. For this reason, spagyric preparations are also suitable for the treatment of patients who lack vitality and elderly patients. Initial aggravation almost never occurs unless one considers particular detoxification reactions to be initial aggravations. With such processes, it would be more reasonable however to talk in terms of reactions.

Spagyric medicine actually pre-dates homoeopathy by about two centuries. Homoeopathy's father, Samuel Hahnemann, abided by the same basic philosophy but differed in execution. Homoeopathic mother tincture, that homoeopaths use, is simply the mercurious level of the plant without the minerals and enzymes found in the salt and sulphur levels. Spagyrics is a branch of medicinal alchemy that enhances the healing properties already existing in plants.

8
The Three Philosophical Principles

Sulphur, mercury, and salt are old alchemical terms. Sulphur doesn't mean here the element, sulphur. Mercury not the element, mercury. And salt not the substance, salt. These substances are used as symbols.

Salt - Mercury – Sulphur

Meanings:

Sulphur stands for soul – astral part

Mercury for life – ether part

Salt for body – physical part

In a spagyric medicament, sulphur, mercury, and salt must be united. Clear parallels to the three levels of substance (salt), information or plan (sulphur) and power (mercury) can be recognized here.

It is indeed the case that in addition to the material basis, which is what makes it possible to handle the remedy in the first place, specific (healing) power must be present to an unlimited extent in spagyric medicaments. Here is the original universal elemental force which has however been modified in accordance with the primary substance. All three substances form a unit. The alchemical term salt denotes among other things the material basis of a spagyric preparation. Mercury in this context stands for the healing power and sulphur for its indication specific orientation.

Spagyrism is, when healing powers are developed from nature which are therapeutically effective when used as medicinal remedies. For alchemy, the metals are cosmic forces transformed into matter, every plant is an accumulator for a particular cosmic-biological force, and spagyrism attempts-based on the alchemical views and knowledge to find these very specific (healing) powers in nature and develop them from the natural substances. For the development of healing powers, various natural substances are subjected to different spagyric preparation methods. We would like to describe a spagyric production method that is perhaps not generally well-known. It is a laboratory process, a special spagyric distillation also called cohobation. This method can be very important at certain stages of medicament production. With the help of cohobation, botanical, mineral, and metallic preparations can be brought onto a higher level of the healing power.

With Cohobation, the solution of a salt, for example, is distilled in a suitable glass apparatus. The distillate obtained in this way is added again to the residue, therefore to the salt which is left behind in the distilling retort. Then distilling is again carried out and the distillate reunited with the residue. A process which from the chemical point of view remains baffling and incomprehensible. This process can be repeated a variable number of times. It leads to a modification of the salt and to a modification of the solvent and distillate. For spagyrism, the most important thing is that this process leads to the development of a highly substance-specific healing power. The solvent is repeatedly separated by distillation from the salt and then united with it again. Here, we again encounter the separation and uniting that give rise to the word, spagyrism. This is a process that one can compare with exhalation and inhalation as described above. What really takes place during cohobation is hard to describe in words. One should witness the preparation process once or have carried it out oneself. By contemplating such a spagyric process one can come closer to intuitively grasping its true nature than is possible based on anything that can be described in words.

So-called rotations and circulations are applied for very similar purposes as cohobation. These are very special spagyric reflux distillations which can also be carried out in accordance with certain rhythms like, for example, the day/night rhythm. These rotations or circulations are carried out over a long period of time (e.g. for 28 days). They too lead to a strong energization and to the development and intensification of the substance-specific healing power.

Additionally, there are the so-called calcinations and reverberations, here energy is always supplied in the form of intense or very intense heat and many other procedures.

The description of a process includes both the method and the substance or substances which are prepared using the method. The therapeutic efficacy of spagyric preparations provides proof of the correctness of the processes.

Spagyric preparations can be very well combined with high-quality waters or with medicinal herb teas. These represent ideal vehicles for the taking of spagyric medicaments. One can, for example, add the patient's entire daily dose of the required spagyric preparation to one litre of water and shake it thoroughly so that the components that are only slightly soluble in water are distributed as homogeneously as possible. The ethereal oils of the medicinal plants are still contained in spagyric preparations. But the concentration of ethereal oils is so small that they become distributed very homogeneously in the water by shaking. The patient is instructed to take these preparations at times distributed throughout the day. The solutions should be freshly prepared every day.

One can also use teas which are produced with a drug mixture suitable for the indication. As a rule, medicinal herb teas are allowed to cool before the spagyric remedy is added.

It is easy for working patients to take such preparations with them in a bottle to take at their place of work.

Spagyrism is an ancient healing art. But it is still important today. And in future, when mankind develops beyond the one-sidedness of the materialistic mode of thought, this importance will become considerably greater.

9

Spagyric Electro-Homoeopathy

Electrohomoeopathy is a nature based therapeutic system becoming increasingly popular now-a-days. Many people are familiar with the plants for their medicinal uses and on increasing number are starting to discover spagyric, a system of natural medicine which has been in existence for more than five hundred years.

Having taken this basic principles of natural healing Theophrastus Paracelsus of Switzerland and Siddhar Nagarjuna prepared spagyric essences from the plants with the help of a natural biochemical media which is the main source of life that is water. And the prepared essences now contains such substances of the plants which have the capacity to enhance organic work, providing nutrients in a more saturated and potentive form for their easy absorption in the body and excretion of waste materials from the body through its natural drainage system.

The method of preparation of the drug is very simple but more scientific in a process called cohobation. The end product of cohobation is designated as spagyric.

The word spagyric is a combination of two Greek words as spa meaning separate and agerio to recombine. In which procedure crude substantial bonds of the plant components diffused to minute particles and after re-combination possesses the properties of the body fluids, containing various bio-electrodes from which the cell as organic unit gets nutrition for its growth development and excretes waste materials for better maintenance.

So those medicines which contains the bio-electrodes of carbohydrates, proteins, fats, herbo minerals and vitamins in a fine absorbable way and become responsible for maintenance for cellular health, having managed the work of cellular absorption and excretion which grossly represents for an organ and as well as for the body. As a result, body maintains the state homoeostesis which condition is called as a physiological healthy condition. Now it is obvious that Eletrohomoeopathy means the word "Electro" represents for the bio-electrodes as cellular nutritive substances which are responsible for maintenance of the state of steadiness (representing for the word Homoeo) and in the suffering body (the pathus).

Absorption of Spagyric Essences

The absorption of a drug involves its passage across cell membrane. The following factors played major role in absorption of the Electrohomoeopathy essences.

Physical State: Mostly essences are liquids so easily absorbed in compare to solids.

Particle Size: Essences are the energetic particles as well as the trace elements and micro-elements so absorbed easily.

Solubility: Essences are in the form of solution, so easily absorbed in compare to solids.

Concentration: Spagyric essences are concentrated form therefore easily absorbed than dilute solution.

The bio-electrodes used in solution are nothing just the nutrients minerals vitamins like supporting ingredient in more active stage for reparation, growth and development of cellular life. Due to high Electrical affinity of solution its application in the nerve points as external applicant, in oral use or of hypodermic injection stimulate the nerves immediately and having mingled with the body fluids try to maintain acid base balance very easily as per the requirement of body if given in right proportion. So efficacy of these remedies are more faster than other and control of disease is more easier in the new therapy.

Safety of Spagyric Medicines

Spagyric medicine are produce in such a way that no alkaloids or toxic molecules can be found in the final products. Though pure and undiluted their efficacy may be compared with the "highly diluted" homoeopathic remedies. They have no known side effects. The advantage of these spagyric essence that it consists therefore the fact that they contain organic and inorganic materials and very well compatible by small alcohol content and the dosage recommended on adherence to normal conditions. The active substances of the essence can be proven with modern analytic technology, both in quality and quantity.

Plant Life Concentrates contain a unique ability to:

1. Alkalise the PH, neutralizing acidity
2. Remove many toxins and toxic molecules out of the body
3. Cleanse and purify the liver
4. Oxygenate the cells, allowing more oxygen into the cells and brain
5. Destroy harmful free radicals
6. Rid body of harmful bacteria
7. Purify and regulate the blood, effecting blood circulation and blood sugar levels
8. Build the immune system
9. Relieve pain caused by acidosis and inflammatory processes

We are far away from the system of similar and the pathogenesy of Hahnemann. It is true that this system is attractive on the intellectual ground, but it is very easy to be lost in it, even for an experienced homoeopath.

The big dilemma, center of homoeopath discussions, is to know if we have to privilege or not a high dilution rather than a low dilution. It is wiped out, as far as spagyric is always turned to the composed and asserts that it is not necessary to dilute a substance to the infinite to increase its field and depth of action. The spagyric experience demonstrates that easily.

This bring us to raise an issue that takes us particularly to heart, the one of mineral elements, which are present as traces in spagyric essence. The presence of these micro nutrients or trace elements (area of the composed) flow directly and specifically from the spagyric way of preparation. Micro-nutrients (Cu, Zn, Si, Mg, etc.) have a considerable action as modifier or corrector of the field, as well on a structural point of view as plastic material, as on a functional point of view as bio-catalyst of enzymatic reaction necessary to any life.

As a matter of fact, the vegetal spagyric elixir is characterized more than any other herbal or homoeopathic pharmaceutical preparation by the extend of its range of action, which is located at three different levels;

1. Symptomatic Level (Sulphur)

Are of action of the herbal medicine and aromatherapy (Allopathy, short time effect and with limited duration in relation with the presence of active principles (alkaloids, flavonoid, terpenes, etc.). However, spagyrists give importance to the problem of "vaporization of salts", formula that constitute in the modern chemistry, a total nonsense, by virtue of the steady character that is peculiar to the saline compound. The processes of salt vaporization constitute in the microcosm.

2. Energetic Level (Mercury)

- Area of action of homoeopathy
- Variable terms of action
- In relation with the vibratory quality of the product and the receptivity of the patient.

3. Structural and Biocatalyst Level (Salt)

- Area of action of micro-nutritionist medicine (micro-nutrients)
- Durable and in depth correction of the field
- Long term effects (several month)
- Reconstitution of the mineral reserves of the organism (Mg, Si, Mn, Cu, Zn, Co, etc.)

This repartition of sulphur, salt and mercury principles on the basis of Paracelsus, is also the foundation of the holistic approach of the patient. Because if the spagyric is interested by the illness as a nosologic entity, it does not neglect to be interested like we have seen in the field that was favorable for the emergence of the illness. Exchange of ions across the cell wall and transmissive actions of the nerves.

When electricity flows into the body from and electro-stimulator and impulse or action potential is evoked in the nerve cells, which is transmitted to the special cord and brain causing the sensation of perception. Even though electricity is not sent by an electrical device, there are many special type of receptor nerve cells which can sent pain, light, sound, taste and soon existing on the surface of the body, in the eyes, ears, tongue, nose, skin and other parts. When each receptor gets various types of stimulation electric impulse is invoked and transmitted to the sensory nerves, reaching the brain through the spinal cords which causes sensation or perception. On the other hand impulse are transmitted retrogressively through another band of nerves called motor nerves to each part of the body muscles, so that arm, leg, eyes and other organs work well. These impulse of the nerves are generated by the instantaneous action of ions moving between inside and outside the nerve cells, nerve fiber the transmits the action. When a nerve is not active (state of response) their many kalium ions (k+) distributed inside each nerve fiber. Many natrium (Na+) ions are distributed outside the cells. This is same as above maintained pattern for cells general when various kinds of stimulations (for example pain, heat, light, sound and taste) are given to the nerve from outside body. The nerves react to them, the character of walls of nerve dells charges and instantaneously numerous natrium ions rush into the nerve cells in the meantime the kalium ions are going out.

At this very moment body loses its electrical balance and voltage (impulse, action potentials) rises instantly, which is transmitted in the wave form to spinal cord through the nerve fiber then to the brain where cause various perception like pain, heat, etc. like this being given some kind of stimulation the character of walls of nerve cells changes with inner and outer ions exchanging places. Thus arises the action potential, which phenomenon is called excitement of nerves. After one excitement is finished natrium comes back in its position. The moment of ions in this restorative stage is caused by nerve cells having spent their naturally energy taking in the pushing out these ions by force. This action is called active transport. Thus the nerve cells generates electricity by moment of ions between nerve fiber.

Electricity in the living body involved directly with the body functions all cells can pass from a state of physiological rest to one of excitation in response to stimuli. Such electrical stimuli helps to excite the tissue, muscle and by which bio-electrical phenomenon in the living body becomes more active.

Bio electrodes used in electrohomeopathy system as spagyric essences helps to balance the body physiology. According to the electrohomeopathic therapy the whole human body is maintained by two opposite types of works conducted inside it. That's the work of absorption and excretion. Such absorption and excretion are conducted by two principal channels inside the body through the fluid media. As we have previously discussed about the work of body fluids for maintenance of body the absorption of nutrients and excretion of material as cag gas. All depends upon a well balanced bioelectrical phenomenon. The acidity and alkalinity two physiochemical condition balance perfectly by well selected diet. Electrohomeopathic herbal specifics are nothing just dietary supplement which contains bio-electrodes of various proportion in a fine well soluble media water. Which carries the bio-electrodes very easily to nook and corner of the body and activate the sluggish organs as well as controls the over functioning of organic work and balance. The bio-electrodes on this way activates certain pathways of circulation and correcting malfunction in absorption, transportation and excretion. By redistributing mineral salts trace elements etc. which due to stress disease or medicine have become locked up in the wrong place. For instance infection and cortisone treatment induce transport of zinc and iron to the liver and the release of copper to the blood stream, conditions or some signal or else may be lacking to restore normal effect. In odema sodium in excess quantity enters the cells. Electrohomoeopathic medicines restores cell membrane integrity and restores proper absorption, transportation and excretion which are essential in accordance with transformation of matter.

By compensating for deficiency induced inactive pathway it means redistributing any scarce elements to the tissues at potential risk or activating some alternative pathway for instance Vitamin E and selenium have a number of overlapping roles, if vitamin E synthesis is stimulated selenium deficiency will be less critical.

Many of our chronic diseases are actually caused due to excessive inflammation. Inflammation is initiated by the neutrophils, it's granules release cytotoxic metabolites aimed at destroying microbials and viral invaders, and by basophils to destroy allergens. Cytotoxic metabolites include peroxides and free radicals, these oxidizing elements can also destroy the fatty acids that comprise cell membranes, causing necrosis of tissues in the inflammated area, their over activity is suppressed by anti-oxidants produced by the cells. Anti-oxidants include the enzymes, vitamins A, E and C, zinc, copper and selenium, hence, these elements are required for the immune system or body's defence mechanism, the inflammatory attack and the healing of tissues. The special aspect of the spagyric technique followed in preparation of Electrohomoeopathy Medicines is that importance is given to the mineral salts which are present in the plants grown in their natural habitats, as plants grown in different environments usually show a wide variation of mineral salt composition.

In Biochemistry, mineral salt preparations are prescribed for therapeutic uses and as Physiologists have established salt-hunger or 'Chelation' causes ailments in human beings. The majority of mineral salts are soluble in water not in alcohol, so, even from the modern scientific view it will not be wrong to say Electro-Homoeopathy is totally Scientific in which mineral salts produced in and from natural sources (In Biochemistry Chemically produced mineral salts are used throughout) in minute form is prescribed to relieve mineral salt deficiency or 'Chelation' in human body, thus to effect a far more natural and specific cure.

10
Energy in the Organism

For the modern day practitioners recognizing the importance of the emergency in bio-energy medicine is vital. Einstein's famous equation $E=MC^2$ mathematically describes how matter and energy are interrelated. Einstein says that matter and energy were in fact two different forms of the same thing. Matter is a manifestation of energy and all vital processes in the living organism are influenced and controlled by electro-magnetic forces. Italian Physist Prof. Carlorubia, who was awarded the 1984 Nobel Prize, stressed that matter only represents a very minute part of universe and that the phenomena of energetic interaction and resonance which control matter are far more important.

Extensive bio-research reveals that all cells in the living organism communicate with each other and have ability to store and emit particles of light which were called bio-photons by the German biophysicist Fritz A. Pop of the University of Kaiserlauten.

As we know body is a composition of number of organs, and organs are the composition of number of tissues, and tissues are formed with the help of number of cells. Which cells are the minute but root particles of the body through which the body receives nutrition and excretes waste materials. Such cellular reception and excretion vitalizes the works of tissues organs as well as the body. Abnormal cellular regeneration and degeneration are two indicative phases of disease condition. These two opposite situations depend upon the two opposite works maintained by the cell. The absorption and excretion. Finally, absorption and excretion of the micro-nutrients occur through a fluid media. The main source of that fluids the blood and in course of time it changes its position to lymph. Such lymph and blood are the basic fluids of the body directly or indirectly responsible for all the happening in the cellular bed.

Cesare Mattie prepared 38 specific remedies from 33 plants/ herbs having classified them in eight groups as No.1– Scrofuloso group containing 12 specifics for lymphatic disorders. No. 2 – Angioticos group containing three specifics for disorders of blood and its circulating channels. No. 3 – Febrifugo group containing two specifics for the motor and sensorial nerve fibers. No. 4 – Canceroso group containing seventeen tissue specifics for structural disorders. No. 5 – Vermifugo group containing two specifics to provide resistance against the micro organisms. No. 6 – The venerio groups containing five specifics as cellular resistance enhancer against the micro organisms. No. 7 – Lymphatic group containing two specifics for their special effects on the lymphoid tissues for production of lymph as well as blood with the immunoglobulins. No. 8 – Pettoralis group of medicines contains nine specifics to control the disorders of respiratory system. Then five fluids called as eletricites like white, blue, red, green & yellow provide their effects on the nerve points to enhance their action and control the organic work with the help of a supportive medicine from other eight groups. Besides these, two other specifics, one is APP for the skin and the another one Slass as a laxative.

1. Eight or ten globules of Scrofoloso dry will render an intoxicated man sober, will stop a threatening of paralysis, or arrest an attack of fainting, etc.

2. Two or three globules of the same remedy on the tongue will restore digestion if it is difficult or arrested, or give appetite and sleep; stop cramp of the stomach, allay toothache, etc.
3. Several spoonfuls of Canceroso, of the first or second dilution, often immediately stop spasmodic contractions of the womb; and by means of this remedy sufficiently continued, all the ailments which trouble a woman during and after confinement can be stopped.
4. Strong compresses of Blue Electricity stop the pain and arrest the flow of blood from a wound, and make it speedily close and heal.
5. Several compresses of White Electricity stop immediately neuralgia in the head; one gargle is often sufficient to stop the most obstinate toothache.
6. A sufficiently prolonged treatment with Scrofoloso, and applications of Electricity will cause the solution and expulsion of a calculus, the closure of a hernia, and will bring back colour and life to chlorotic patients.
7. Fevers and liver diseases may be stamped out by Febrifugo, internally, and functions of Febrifugo novo.

These are experiments which beginners may make in order to prove the surprising efficacy of the Electro-Homoeopathic medicines.

It is very generally supposed that confidence of faith is necessary in order to feel the good effects of the remedies; Oppositions say that this is the secret of homoeopathy. It cannot be side with regard to medicine that faith suffices. Can it be faith or confidence which cures the suckling infant who has no other medicines but those which are given through the nurse? What faith can an intoxicated man, a person in a fainting fit, a madman, have, who are nevertheless cured? Doubtless confidence is necessary, but not that the effect of the remedy may be obtained, but that the prescribed course may be carried out with sincerity and intelligence. Faith is also necessary especially for beginners, in order to induce them not to put too many globules in the glass, seeing they are so small; there must be confidence that the patient may persevere for the time necessary to secure the result, to avoid the temptation to grasp after a more rapid cure by the use of stronger doses. Confidence is only necessary at the commencement; once the results are seen, conviction and certainty follow.

The development of the complex remedy systems established today did not run in a straight line. Different starting points led to different healing systems, e.g.,

The humoral pathological way of thinking,

Spagyrics based on Paracelsus,

Electro Homoeopathy by Mattei.

Advantages of Electrohomoeopathy

1. It is holistic, pure herbal healing system.
2. Vitiation of blood & lymph is root cause of the disease.
3. Cohobation is a specific manufacturing procedure by which the medicines as a spagyric essence provide nutritions to the cells.
4. Spagyric essence are non-poisonous, non-metallic, synthetic materials.
5. The therapeutic system always respects natural healing principle as believed.
6. Remedies are cheaper, safer and quicker.
7. There are no contra indications or interaction between any other remedies so far.
8. Economic use of raw drug materials help for long preservation of natural herbarium.

9. Both acute and chronic diseases are managed/cared in a natural way by enhancing the immunity of the body that is purifying blood and lymph.
10. Drug proving in electrohomoeopathy emphasized on diseased body because organism are more sensitive than the healthy body as compared to diseased body.
11. Remedies should not be given to remove the symptoms of disease but to work on the cause of the disease.
12. Those remedies can be used internally as oral pills (globules), drops in water, syrup-based and injections intra-muscular for quick action.
13. Externally these remedies can be used as ointment, lotions, lineaments and compress.
14. These remedies absorbed in the body quicker as it is aqua based.

11

Herbal Medicine

Herbal medicine is also called botanical medicine or phyto-medicine which refers to using a plant's seeds, berries, roots, leaves, bark, or flowers for medicinal purposes. Herbalism has a long tradition of use outside of conventional medicine. It is becoming more mainstream as improvements in analysis and quality control along with advances in clinical research show the value of herbal medicine in the treating and preventing disease.

History of Herbal Medicine

Plants had been used for medicinal purposes long before recorded history. Ancient Chinese and Egyptian papyrus writings describe medicinal uses for plants. Indigenous cultures (such as African and Native American) used herbs in their healing rituals, while others developed traditional medical systems (such as Ayurveda and Traditional Chinese Medicine) in which herbal therapies were used. Researchers found that people in different parts of the world tended to use the same or similar plants for the same purposes.

In the early 19th century, when chemical analysis first became available, scientists began to extract and modify the active ingredients from plants. Later, chemists began making their own version of plant compounds, and over time, the use of herbal medicines declined in favor of drugs.

World Health Organization estimated that 80% of people worldwide rely on herbal medicines for some part of their primary health care. In Germany, about 600-700 plant- based medicines are available and are prescribed by some 70% of German physicians. In the last 20 years in the United States, public dissatisfaction with the cost of prescription medications, combined with an interest in returning to natural or organic remedies, has led to an increase in herbal medicine use.

In many cases, scientists aren't sure what specific ingredient in a particular herb works to treat a condition or illness. Whole herbs contain many ingredients, and they may work together to produce a beneficial effect. Many factors determine how effective an herb will be. For example, the type of environment (climate, bugs, soil quality) in which a plant grew will affect it, as will how and when it was harvested and processed.

The use of herbal supplements has increased dramatically over the past 30 years. Herbal supplements are classified as dietary supplements by the U.S. Dietary Supplement Health and Education Act of 1994. That means herbal supplements unlike prescription drugs can be sold without being tested to prove that they are safe and effective. However, herbal supplements must be made according to good manufacturing practices.

The most commonly used herbal supplements in the U.S. include echinacea (Echinacea purpurea and related species), St. John's wort (Hypericum perforatum), ginkgo (Ginkgo biloba), garlic (Allium sativum), saw palmetto (Serenoa repens), ginseng (Panax ginseng, or Asian ginseng; and Panax quinquefolius, or American ginseng), goldenseal (Hydrastis canadensis), valerian (Valeriana officinalis), chamomile (Matricaria recutita), feverfew (Tanacetum parthenium), ginger (Zingiber officinale), evening primrose (Oenothera biennis), and milk thistle (Silybum marianum).

Often, herbs may be used together because the combination is more effective and may have fewer side effects. Health care providers must take many factors into account when recommending herbs, including the species and variety of the plant, the plant's habitat, how it was stored and processed, and whether or not there are contaminants (including heavy metals and pesticides).

Herbal medicine is used to treat many conditions, such as asthma, eczema, premenstrual syndrome, rheumatoid arthritis, migraine, menopausal symptoms, chronic fatigue, and irritable bowel syndrome, among others. Herbal supplements are best taken under the guidance of a trained health care provider. Be sure to consult with your doctor or pharmacist before taking any herbs. Some common herbs and their uses are discussed below.

Ginkgo (Ginkgo biloba) has been used in traditional medicine to treat circulatory disorders and enhance memory. Although not all studies agree, ginkgo may be especially effective in treating dementia (including Alzheimer's disease) and intermittent claudication (poor circulation in the legs). It also shows promise for enhancing memory in older adults. Laboratory studies have shown that ginkgo improves blood circulation by dilating blood vessels and reducing the stickiness of blood platelets. By the same token, this means ginkgo may also increase the effect of some blood-thinning medications, including aspirin. People taking blood-thinning medications should ask their doctor before using ginkgo.

Kava kava (Piper methysticum) is said to elevate mood, well-being, and contentment, and produce a feeling of relaxation. Several studies have found that kava may be useful in the treatment of anxiety, insomnia, and related nervous disorders. However, there is serious concern that kava may cause liver damage. It's not clear whether the kava itself caused liver damage in a few people or whether it was taking kava in combination with other drugs or herbs. It's also not clear whether kava is dangerous at previously recommended doses, or only at higher doses.

Saw palmetto (Serenoa repens) is used by more than 2 million men in the United States for the treatment of benign prostatic hyperplasia (BPH), a non-cancerous enlargement of the prostate gland. A number of studies suggest that the herb is effective for treating symptoms, including too-frequent urination, having trouble starting or maintaining urination, and needing to urinate during the night.

St. John's wort (Hypericum perforatum) is well known for its antidepressant effects. In general, most studies have shown that St. John's wort may be an effective treatment for mild to moderate depression, and has fewer side effects than most other prescription anti-depressants. But the herb interacts with a wide variety of medications, including birth control pills, so it is important to take it only under the guidance of a herbal medicine practitioner.

Valerian (Valeriana officinalis) is a popular alternative to commonly prescribed medications for sleep problems because it is considered to be both safe and gentle. Some studies indicated, although not all have found valerian to be effective. Unlike many prescription sleeping pills, valerian may have fewer side effects such as morning drowsiness.

Echinacea preparations (from Echinacea purpurea and other Echinacea species) may improve the body's natural immunity. Echinacea is one of the most commonly used herbal products, but studies are mixed as to whether it can help prevent or treat colds. Analysis of clinical studies examining the effect of Echinacea on the incidence and duration of the common cold found that Echinacea supplements decreased the odds of getting a cold by 58%. It also shortened the duration of a cold by 1.4 days.

Buying standardized herbal supplements helps ensure you will get the right dose and the effects similar to human clinical trials. Consult a doctor or pharmacist about which herbal supplements are the best choice for your health concerns.

When used correctly, herbs can help treat a variety of conditions and in some cases may have fewer side effects than some conventional medications. But because they are unregulated, herbal products are often mislabeled and may contain additives and contaminants that aren't listed on the label. Some herbs may cause allergic reactions or interact with conventional drugs, and some are toxic if used improperly or at high doses. Taking herbs on your own increases your risk, so it is important to consult your doctor or pharmacist before taking herbal medicines. Some examples of adverse reactions from certain popular herbs are described below.

St. John's wort can cause your skin to be more sensitive to the sun's ultraviolet rays, and may cause an allergic reaction, stomach upset, fatigue, and restlessness. Clinical studies have found that St. John's wort also interferes with the effectiveness of many drugs, including the blood thinner warfarin (Couamdin), protease inhibitors for HIV, birth control pills, certain asthma drugs, and many other medications. In addition, St. John's wort should not be taken with prescribed anti-depressant medication.

Kava kava has been linked to liver toxicity. Kava has been taken off the market in several countries.

Valerian may cause sleepiness, and in some people it may even have the unexpected effect of overstimulating instead of sedating.

Garlic, ginkgo, fever-few, and ginger, among other herbs, may increase the risk of bleeding.

Evening primrose (Oenothera biennis) may increase the risk of seizures in people who have seizure disorders.

Some herbal supplements, especially those imported from Asian countries, may contain high levels of heavy metals, including lead, mercury, and cadmium. It is important to purchase herbal supplements from reputable manufacturers to ensure quality. Talk to your health care provider for more information.

Nearly one-third of Americans use herbs. Unfortunately, a study in the New England Journal of Medicine found that nearly 70% of people taking herbal medicines (most of whom were well educated and had a higher-than-average income) were reluctant tell their doctors that they used complementary and alternative medicine. Many herbs can interact with prescription medications and cause unwanted or dangerous reactions. Be sure to consult your doctor before trying any herbal products.

The herbs available in most stores come in several different forms: teas, syrups, oils, liquid extracts, tinctures, and dry extracts (pills or capsules). Teas can be made from dried herbs left to soak for a few minutes in hot water, or by boiling herbs in water and then straining the liquid. Syrups, made from concentrated extracts and added to sweet-tasting preparations, are often used for sore throats and coughs. Oils are extracted from plants and often used as rubs for massage, either by themselves or as part of an ointment or cream. Tinctures and liquid extracts are made of active herbal ingredients dissolved in a liquid (usually water, alcohol, or glycerol). Tinctures are typically a 1:5 or 1:10 concentration, meaning that one part of the herb is prepared with five to ten parts (by weight) of the liquid. Liquid extracts are more concentrated than tinctures and are typically a 1:1 concentration. A dry extract form is the most concentrated form of a herbal product.

Currently, no organization or agency regulates the manufacture or certifies the labeling of herbal preparations. This means you can't be sure that the amount of the herb contained in the bottle, or even from dose to dose, is the same as what is stated on the label. Some herbal preparations are standardized, meaning that the preparation is guaranteed to contain a specific amount of the active ingredients of the herb.

However, it is still important to ask companies making standardized herbal products about their product's guarantee. It is important to sought professional advice or see an expert in herbal medicine about the recommended doses of any herbal products.

Herbalists, chiropractors, naturopathic physicians, pharmacists, medical doctors, and practitioners of Traditional Chinese Medicine all may use herbs to treat illness. Naturopathic physicians believe that the body is continually striving for balance and that natural therapies can support this process.

In some countries in Europe unlike the U.S. herbs are classified as drugs and are regulated. The German Commission E, an expert medical panel, actively researches their safety and effectiveness.

While still not widely accepted, herbal medicine is being taught more in medical schools and pharmacy schools. More health care providers are learning about the positive and potentially negative effects of using herbal medicines to help treat health conditions. Some health care providers, including doctors and pharmacists, are trained in herbal medicine. They can help people create treatment plans that use herbs, conventional medications and lifestyle changes to promote health.

In the conventional system of herbal medicine, the medicines are prepared in numerous ways. The methods keep on varying depending on the nature of the herbs those are being used.

Most of these methods comprise of decoctions (boiled teas), infusions (hot teas), and tinctures (alcohol and water extracts). There are other methods also which include making hot baths taken by the patients, steam inhalation of several herbal plants and finally aromatherapy.

Below some of the methods of preparing herbal medicines are described:

Aloe Vera

Medicinal Parts: The yellow juice taken out from the inner skin of leaves and the gel from the leaves.

Method of Preparation: This is very simple you need to tear a lower leaf and apply to the wound directly. Aloe is widely applied in several skin conditions.

Medicinal Parts: Leaves

Method of Preparation: It is used as a tranquilizer. To treat injuries, make a hot squash using 2 teaspoons of these leaves in one cup of hot water. Boil the mixture for 10 minutes. Then apply it with a clean cloth.

Berberry

Medicinal Parts: Bark of the root

Method of Preparation: You need to boil the bark in water and then squeeze the pulp. Administer the pulp on the affected area.

Bookoo

Medicinal Parts: Leaves

Method of Preparation: You need to add those leaves into hot teas that is called as infusion.

Carum

Medicinal Parts: Seeds

Method of Preparation: Mix fresh seeds into food or chew it a teaspoonful at a time. After crushing the seeds you can prepare an infusion of it.

Cascara

Medicinal Parts: Dried and aged bark

Method of Preparation: For preparing the medicine you need to store the bark for a year because the fresh bark holds chemicals which can cause serious intestinal cramps.

Guidelines for Preparation of Herbal Medicines

Lack of standardization can cause differences among certain products. So the raw material you are using must be standardized.

Make it sure that you are not using larger than the recommended dose.

In traditional herbal medicine systems, herbal remedies are prepared in several rather standardized ways which usually vary based upon the plant utilized, and sometimes, what condition is being treated. Some of these methods include: infusions (hot teas), decoctions (boiled teas), tinctures (alcohol and water extracts), and macerations (cold-soaking) which are detailed more fully herein. In indigenous Indian medicine systems, medicine men or shamans generally use these same methods in addition to others. Others include preparing plants in hot baths (in which the patient is soaked in it or bathed with it), inhalation of powdered plants (like snuff), steam inhalation of various aromatic plants boiled in hot water, and even aromatherapy. The well trained herbalist will always thoroughly review the time-honored method in which a plant has been traditionally prepared it holds important information for preparing an effective herbal remedy.

The biological or therapeutic activity of a medicinal plant is closely related to the plant chemicals in it. These chemicals can be classified into major groups of chemicals such as essential oils, alkaloids, acids, steroids, tannins, saponins and so forth. Each one of these classes of chemicals may have a preferred effective method of extraction which facilitates getting the chemicals out of the plant and into the herbal remedy that is being prepared. For example, some active chemicals found in plants are not soluble or dissolved in water, therefore just preparing a hot tea with the plant, or even boiling the plant in hot water won't extract these chemicals into the resulting water extract/tea remedy. Generally, if they aren't water soluble, they won't be broken down in the digestive process either, so taking the plant in capsules or tablets won't be much help either. If the active chemicals aren't in the prepared remedy-then it probably won't provide any benefits that are attributed to these chemicals. These same chemicals may however be more soluble in alcohol which is why the time-honored method of preparing the plant has been as a tincture (or a water/alcohol extract).

Interestingly, this is also the reason why some plants are prepared in one manner to treat one specific condition, yet are prepared in a different way to treat a completely different condition. For example; preparing an infusion/tea of a plant might extract a delicate group of anti-inflammatory plant steroids to treat arthritis (and leave behind other non-water soluble chemicals). Yet when the same plant is prepared in alcohol as a tincture, the delicate steroids are degraded or burned-up in the alcohol but different antibacterial alkaloids (which are only soluble in alcohol) are extracted instead. This may explain why a tea of the plant is used for arthritis while a tincture of the same plant is traditionally used to treat various bacterial infections.

The rainforest shaman or rural herbal healer is not a trained chemist with high-tech machines and scientific instruments at their disposal to isolate and study plant chemicals. Their knowledge has been built over time, decades of passed down empirical knowledge from trial and error, human experimentation, and even destiny, about the best way to prepare medicinal plants into effective herbal remedies. Yet, more often times than not, plant chemists and scientists generally get around to verifying that these so-called "uneducated" herbal healers have manouvered through complex chemical differences, reactions and interactions, and different types of chemicals "unwittingly" developing the most efficient manner to extract and utilize their biological activities. It is usually the shaman's knowledge, however, that the really smart scientists start with which gives specific clues as to which types of chemicals might be present in a plant based upon the traditional preparation method used.

The first step in producing a herbal medicine is sourcing the good raw plant materials. Ensure about their harvesting practices. Instructions for the main preparation methods used in the reference guides and in the main plant section are as follows.

Infusions

Infusions are typically used for delicate herbs, leaves and fresh tender plants. Preparing an infusion is much like making a cup of tea. Water is brought just to a boil and then poured over an herb (or combination of herbs), it is covered and allowed to sit/steep for 10-15 minutes or so. It can be prepared in the drinking cup (by just pouring the heated water over the herb in the cup) or by dropping the herb into the pot which the water was heated in. Empty gauze tea-bags are even available at some herb stores which can be filled with herbs and then sealed with iron. If an infusion is prepared in the heating pan/pot, it's best to use a ceramic pot with a lid (avoid metal pots). Stirring it a few times while steeping (especially with cut herbs) is helpful. Keeping the infusion covered while steeping is generally recommended as well (place a saucer on top of the cup, or a lid on top of the pot). The ratio of herb to water can vary depending on the remedy, the plant, and whether cut herb or powdered herb is used. Generally using 1 teaspoon of powdered herb or 2 teaspoons of more bulky cut herb in a 6-8 ounce cup of water is sufficient. If using a powdered herb; stir once halfway through the seeping time and let the powder settle to the bottom of the cup, then drink the infusion off the top (leaving the sediment in the bottom of the cup). If using a cut herb, strain the infusion with a tea-strainer after seeping. Infusions are best prepared as needed and taken the same day it was prepared and can be taken hot, warm, or cold. Standard dosages of infusions are generally one teacup (6-8 ounces), two or three times daily. The entire day's dosage can be prepared in the morning (2-3 cups at one time), and the remainder refrigerated until ready to use. The exceptions are the more aromatic plants with active essential oils. These are best prepared in single dosages (by the cupful) as needed and taken immediately (and while still hot/warm).

Decoctions

Decoctions are usually the method of choice when working with tougher and more fibrous plants, barks and roots (and which have water soluble chemicals). Instead of just steeping it in hot water, the plant material is boiled for a longer period of time to soften the harder woody material and release its active constituents. To prepare a decoction, select a ceramic pot with a snug fitting lid. Measure the amount of herb needed (usually the same ratio of 1 teaspoon powdered herb or 2 teaspoons of cut herb per 8 ounces of water) into the pot and add the proper amount of cold water depending on how many cups of the decoction you wish to prepare. Turn on the heat to medium high and bring to a roiling boil. Place the lid on the pot and reduce the heat to medium or medium-low so that the mixture stays at a good simmer. Simmer it covered for 20 minutes. If you can see steam escaping or smell the aroma of the herb, your lid is not tight enough and valuable essential oils are escaping. After 20 minutes, remove from heat and cool slightly. If using cut herbs, strain the mixture through a tea strainer into a teacup. When straining, make sure to press on the cut herb pieces in the strainer to get as much liquid/ decoction out of the herb pieces as possible. If using powdered herb, allow the powder to settle to the bottom of the pot and then pour off the decoction from the top into a teacup (any sediment missed will settle to the bottom of the teacup). Standard dosages for decoction are generally one-half to one cup, two or three times daily. Again, the entire day's dosage can be prepared in the morning (2-3 cups at one time), and the remainder refrigerated until ready to use later in the day.

Strong Decoctions

Depending on the type of plant material used, strong decoctions are prepared in two general ways. The first involves boiling the mixture longer. This is usually indicated when working with larger woody pieces of bark. Longer boiling time, up to 2 hours or more, is sometimes necessary to break down, soften, and extract the larger pieces. Alternatively, when smaller woody pieces are used yet a stronger remedy is wanted, the decoction is prepared as above (boiling 20 minutes), then it is allowed to soak overnight before straining out the herb. When straining, again, make sure to press on the cut herb pieces in the strainer to get as much moisture/decoction out of the herb pieces.

Tinctures

A tincture is an alcohol and water extract which is used when plants have active chemicals that are not very soluble in water, and/or when a larger quantity is prepared for convenience and wanted for longer term storage. Many properly prepared plant tinctures can last several years or more without losing potency. The percentage of alcohol usually helps determine its shelf-life: the more alcohol used, the longer the shelf life. Sometimes the percentage of alcohol and water is unique to the herbs that are used as some active ingredients are more soluble in alcohol and others more soluble in water. The type of alcohol can vary from vodka, rum, or 90 to 180 proof grain alcohol In the Amazon, a sugar-cane alcohol resembling rum and called aguardiente is often used to prepare plant tinctures and it is 40 to 50% alchohol (or 80 to 90 proof).

To prepare a tincture with a shelf-life of at least one year, plan on using a minimum of 40% alcohol (so you can extract an herb in a bottle of 80 proof vodka or rum without adding any water). Use a clean glass bottle or jar with tight fitting lid or cork. Use a dark colored bottle (like a recycled green/amber wine bottle) or plan on storing the bottle out of the sunlight. When working with dried plants, use two ounces of plant material (cut or powder) for every 8 ounces (1 cup) of liquid. Since many cut herbs can be bulky, measure the amount of cut herb by weight and not volume (i.e.; most cooks would tell you 2 tablespoons of butter is 1 ounce... however a lightweight bulky leaf is not as heavy as butter in the same volume or by the tablespoon). A "standard 4:1 tincture" usually means 1 part herb to 4 parts liquid (or as above, 1 ounce herb to 4 ounces of liquid). To prepare approximately 1 cup of tincture (some of the liquid will be absorbed by the dry plant material) place 2 ounces of the herb (cut up or powdered) into your clean glass container. Pour ½ cup (4 ounces) of distilled water and ½ cup (4 ounces) of 180 proof alcohol into the container (or just use 1 cup of straight 80 proof vodka and no water). Seal the container and store at room temperature away from direct sunlight. Shake the bottle/jar at least once daily while allowing it to soak/extract for at least two weeks (larger woody cut herb pieces may need to soak for 4 weeks). At the end of two weeks, filter the tincture through a strainer to remove the plant parts (pressing hard on the plant material to get as much liquid out as possible) and pour into a fresh clean glass container and seal. Some like to pour it through a cheese cloth and then use the cheese cloth to more easily wring out the liquid from the plant material. If using a powdered plant for the tincture, stop shaking for three days and the powder will settle to the bottom. Pour the tincture off the top through a piece of cheesecloth to filter it.

Since this method uses a higher ratio of plant to liquid and helps concentrate the chemicals through the use of alcohol, dosages needed for tinctures are usually much less than infusions and decoctions. Average dosages for tinctures are about 1-2 millilitres (about 30 to 60 drops) two to three times daily. The tincture can be placed directly in the mouth for immediate absorption, or placed in a small amount of water or juice. If you dislike the alcohol content (or want to give the remedy to a child), place the dosage in about 1-2 ounces of very hot water and most of the alcohol will be evaporated in the hot water in a minute or two. Store the tincture at room temperature and away from direct sunlight.

Macerations

This method of preparation is certainly the easiest. The fresh or dried plant material is simply covered in cool water and soaked overnight. The herb is strained out and the liquid is taken. Normally this is used for very tender plants and/or fresh plants, or those with delicate chemicals that might be harmed by heating or which might be degraded in strong alcohol. This is also the easiest to adapt to western methods, since tablets or capsules can be used instead. Alternatively, just stir the ground plant powder into juice, water or smoothies and drink.

Poultices and Compresses

Many herbal remedies are applied directly to the skin as poultices usually on rashes and wounds and as topical pain relieving remedies. Poultices are prepared in various ways... from the jungle shaman chewing up fresh leaves or roots and spitting them out onto the skin, to mashing up fresh leaves or roots by hand or with a mortar and pestle. Sometimes just enough hot water is poured over dried or fresh plant material to soften them. Then the wet herbs are placed directly on the skin or between two pieces of cloth and laid on the skin. A light cotton bandage to bind the poultice to the area is generally used (or in the jungle, a nice large flexible leaf is commonly employed and tied with a bit of twine). Compresses are simply soaking a cloth in a prepared infusion, tincture or decoction and laying the cloth onto the affected part of the body/skin. Since most American readers of this book will only have access to dried plant materials to work with, using compresses instead of poultices will suffice for many of the describe indigenous poultice remedies. More specific adaptations and directions where applicable are found in the main plant section under "Traditional Remedy" where it might say to apply an infusion or decoction topically.

Baths and Bathing Remedies

Quite a few popular jungle remedies which have been used for thousands of years in the Amazon are prepared as vapor baths, or medicinal plants are added to bath water and the patient is soaked in it. This method is not unlike some of the currently evolving dermal delivery systems for drug absorption being employed in conventional medicine. The skin is a wonderful organ capable of absorbing plant chemicals (and even synthetic chemicals) directly through the skin, and into the underlying fat tissue, then into the bloodstream. Since fresh plants are generally used for bathing remedies (chopped or crushed first before adding to the bath water), western adaptations are not always possible when only dried plant materials are available here. In the alternative, try 20 to 30 ounces of a strong decoction or infusion added to your bath water and soak in it for at least 10 minutes.

Tips on Handling Medicinal Plants/Herbs

Insist for herbs that are grown organically, without chemicals and pesticides.

Medicinal parts of plants are best harvested on sunny mornings. Avoid picking leaves, fruits or nuts during and after heavy rainfall.

Leaves, fruits, flowers or nuts must be mature before harvesting. Less medicinal substances are found on young parts.

After harvesting, if drying is required, it is advisable to dry the plant parts either in the oven or air-dried on screens above ground and never on concrete floors.

Store plant parts in sealed plastic bags or brown bottles in a cool dry place without sunlight preferably with a moisture absorbent material like charcoal. Leaves and other plant parts that are prepared properly, well-dried and stored can be used up to six months.

Tips on Preparation for Intake of Herbal Medicines

Use only half the dosage prescribed for fresh parts like leaves when using dried parts.

Do not use stainless steel utensils when boiling decoctions. Only use earthen, enamelled, glass or alike utensils.

As a rule, when boiling leaves and other plant parts, do not cover the pot, and boil in low flame.

Decoctions loose potency after some time. Dispose of decoctions after one day. To keep fresh during the day, keep lukewarm in a flask or thermos.

Always consult with a doctor if symptoms persist or if any sign of allergic reaction develops.

Extraction

Extraction is a process whereby the desired constituents of a plant are removed using a solvent. The following section describes several methods used for preparing extracts, including organic solvent extraction, supercritical gas extraction, and steam distillation.

Organic Solvent Extraction: Organic solvent extraction is one process for separating the desired substance from plant material. As was previously mentioned, dried plants are usually used for extraction, although fresh plants are sometimes used. The plants are first ground and then thoroughly mixed with a solvent such as hexane, benzene, or toluene inside a tank. The choice of solvent depends on several factors including the characteristics of the constituents being extracted, cost, and environmental issues. If the end product will contain trace amounts of residual solvent, a non-toxic solvent must be used. Once the solvent dissolves the desired substances of the plant, it is called "miscella." The miscella is then separated from the plant material (Hornok, 1992). There are a number of techniques for solvent extraction, which include maceration, percolation, and counter-current extraction. The following is a brief description of each.

Maceration: This method involves soaking and agitating the solvent and plant materials together. The solvent is then drained off. Remaining miscella is removed from the plant material through pressing or centrifuging. This method does not totally extract the active ingredients from the plant materials.

Percolation: With this method, the plant material is moistened with solvent and allowed to swell before being placed in one of a series of percolation chambers. The material is repeatedly rinsed with solvent until all the active ingredient has been removed. Solvent is reused until it is saturated. New solvent is used on plant material that is almost completely exhausted, and then re-used on subsequently less exhausted batches. This method is more effective at removing active ingredients than the maceration technique.

Counter-current extraction: This is a highly effective process whereby solvent flows in the opposite direction to plant material. Unlike maceration and percolation, which are batch processes, this method is continuous. Screw extractors and carousel extractors are two types of equipment used for counter-current extraction (Wijesekera, 1991).

Purification and Concentration of Miscella: Miscella that has been separated from the plant material generally contains some unwanted substances such as tannins, pigments, microbial contaminants, or residual solvent. Methods such as decanting, filtration, sedimentation, centrifuging, heating, adsorption, precipitation, and ion exchange are used to separate impurities from the miscella. Sometimes the miscella resulting from solvent extraction is used as the final dosage form. This is known as a "fluid extract" (List and Schmidt, 1989). The miscella is sometimes concentrated in order to increase the proportion of the desired substance. This is done through evaporation or vaporization. Solvent is generally recovered and reused (List and Schmidt, 1989). The degree of concentration depends on the desired end product. Equipment for concentrating the miscella may include descending film, thin layer or plate concentrators. Any method used to concentrate the miscella must avoid excessive heat because the active compounds may be subject to degradation (Wijesekera, 1991).

Sometimes extracts are dried completely using vacuum freeze dryers, cabinet vacuum dryers, continuously operating drum or belt dryers, microwave ovens, or atomizers. The technique for drying depends on the stability of the product and the amount of moisture that must be removed. The resulting powdered extract is less subject to microbial contamination than are liquid extracts (Hornok, 1992).

Extraction with Supercritical Gases: This is a method for extracting active ingredients using gases. The plant material is placed in a vessel that is filled with a gas under controlled temperature and high pressure. The gas dissolves the active ingredients within the plant material, then passes into a separating chamber where both pressure and temperature are lower. The extract precipitates out and is removed through a valve at the bottom of the chamber. The gas is then reused. Gases suitable for supercritical extraction include carbon dioxide, nitrogen, methane, ethane, ethylene, nitrous oxide, sulfur dioxide, propane, propylene, ammonia, and sulfur hexafluoride. An advantage of supercritical extraction is that it can take place at low temperature, thus preserving the quality of temperature-sensitive components (List and Schmidt, 1989).

Steam Distillation

Steam distillation is another method for extracting active ingredients from medicinal plants. The plant material is loaded onto perforated plates inside a cylindrical tank or still, and steam is injected from below. The steam dissolves the desired substances in the plant, then enters a condenser where it is condensed back into a liquid. This condensate then passes into a flask, where the extract either rises to the top or settles to the bottom and is separated from the water. Distillation is complete when there is no more extract present in the condensate. The water may be reused, and the extract is purified through centrifuging and filtering (Hornok, 1992). Other Minor Extraction Methods. Other minor methods for making extracts include cold pressing and the enfleurage process.

Cold pressing is a process used to extract essential oils from citrus plants through pressing (Hornok, 1992). The enfleurage process(to capture the fragrant compounds exuded by plants) is the same as the technique used to make perfume from flowers: purified fats are used to extract essential oils from plant parts. Plant material is spread onto sheets of purified fat, which dissolve the essential oils (List and Schmidt, 1989). Sometimes practitioners of herbal medicine prepare extracts for immediate use. These include aqueous extracts known as decoctions, infusions, or macerations. Plant material is mixed, agitated, and soaked in water to dissolve the active ingredients. Controlling microbial contamination can be difficult in aqueous extracts.

Oily drug extracts, also called "medicinal oils," may be prepared by soaking or macerating the plant material in an oil such as almond, peanut, olive, poppy seed, apricot kernel, or peach kernel oil. Vinegar is sometimes used to extract active ingredients as well. Plant materials are soaked in acetic acid, and the vinegar is consumed as the final dosage form (List and Schmidt, 1989).

Controlling the Quality of Extracts

Once an extract has been produced by one of the methods mentioned above, producers can use a number of tests to evaluate the quality and purity of their product. First, they may examine the physical characteristics of the extract. This may include evaluating its appearance, pH, solubility, total solids content, ash content, and in the case of dried extracts, particle size. Next, they may analyze the components of the extract to be certain it contains the appropriate quantities of desired ingredients. Chromatography (including thin layer, column, high pressure liquid, and gas chromatography) may be used for this. Finally, they may test the extract for impurities such as residual solvents, herbicides, and pesticides and for microbial contamination (Wijesekera, 1991).

Some extracts are labeled and sold as standardized extracts. According to industry sources, the desired constituents in standardized extracts are measured and are listed as a percentage of the total weight of the extract. For example, echinacosides are the desired compounds present in echinacea extract. A capsule containing 250 mg of echinacea extract standardized to 4 percent would contain 10 mg of echinacosides. In some cases, the desired constituent is a known active ingredient.

In cases where the active ingredient has not been identified, another "marker" compound, or substance that is known to be present in the plant, may be measured for the purpose of standardization. Spectrophotometric testing and high pressure liquid chromatography may be used to measure standardized constituents (Standardized Extract Product Guide, 1997).

12

Spiritual Alchemy

"Man is not body. The heart, the spirit, is man. And this spirit is an entire star, out of which, he is built. If therefore a man is perfect in his heart, nothing in the whole light of Nature is hidden from him."

—Paracelsus

According to Chakra healing, any imbalances that exist within any chakra may have profound effects upon either our physical or emotional bodies and by using quartz crystals or gemstones all our chakra centers are balanced back to normalcy and once the chakras have been properly balanced then our body will gradually become disease free, whereas in Hindu or Buddhist tantra specific colors of chakras are awakened through sacred process of spiritual enlightenment to attain the eternal bliss. The word chakra is derived from the Sanskrit word meaning "wheel". Spiritual teachers perceive chakras as colorful wheels or flowers with a hub in the center. The Chakras begin at the base of the spine and finish at the top of the head. Though fixed in the central spinal column they are located on both the front and back of the body, and work through it.

Good health and well-being is achieved when the energy in these chakra centers are balanced. Any blockage or imbalance in these centers results in disease conditions. The use of color can help to restore vitality to the etheric body through the projection of specific color rays, which are then absorbed by the chakra centers. The pituitary gland transforms these colors into revitalizing energies that help rebuild the centers that lack energy. The entire spectrum of colors is derived from sunlight. In the light spectrum, each color vibrates at a different frequency. The vibrations of colors transmit energy, which is used to balance the body's energy centers or chakras.

Every cell in the body requires light energy. Nature itself is full of color. Therefore, it is no surprise that we are drawn to color. Color is energy. The energy vibration of color is used to enhance and balance the physical, emotional and spiritual state of a person.

Harmonious, soothing colors and color combinations are used to promote health and inner harmony, key triggers for healing. The energy of color impacts our mood, health, and thought process. When we heighten our awareness to the energy of color through spiritual or tantric processes, it helps to transform our pattern of health and well being. Importantly, the mood-enhancing properties of color help to improve overall quality of life.

In the teaching of sacred Sanskrit healers, we can find reference to an energy system known as chakras. (Chakra is a Sanskrit word meaning wheel of light.) These vital points in the energy body vibrate at specific color frequencies. Focused color healing works with these points. This is how the use of color can return the body to a vital harmonious system.

Imbalance in the energy centers is thought to be the key reason behind the manifestation of disease. Imbalance, which could occur in the physical, emotional, spiritual and mental levels, is rectified with color therapy.

Colors are light energy at certain wavelengths. This energy is translated into color by the photoreceptors in the retina, called cones. Colors have a direct influence on our thoughts, moods and behaviors because when the energy & color enters our bodies, it stimulates the pituitary and pineal glands to secrete certain hormones. It is said that red color stimulates Our consciousness, emotions and apprehension influence our neuro-immuno-endocrine system. In several traditional medicines, incl. Ayurveda, Homeopathy and Acupuncture disease is considered to originate as a disruption of the life force or the core information matrix. If there is a disorder in the information level, diseases will occur. Inhuman body brain is the core information matrix. Everything in our universe is inter-connected by information-subtle-energy wave fields. Owing to the arrangement in space, each cell knows what is happening to the other cell. The human development in the womb starts with a single cell. How does it know that it needs to develop? Information thus can be placed and shared or transmitted on the energy wave.

Any imbalance of the life force comes from well within our own consciousness. Health could be obtained by removing the distracted information level or consciousness.

The psychological phenomena are the total of the emotional, thought, connection and spiritual emotions. The changes and events in these worlds are projected onto our somatic body (Sigmund Freud, Carl Gustav Jung).

The cell is the basic structural and functional unit of all known living organisms. It is the smallest unit of life that is classified as a living thing, and is often called the 'building block of life'. The Pineal Gland is often referred to as the seat of the spirit or the central level or state of consciousness. According to the Indian Spiritual Chakra system, the pineal gland is part of the physical system corresponding to the Ajna or third eye chakra which can be viewed as a platform where all consciousness meets. The seat of the spirit is the Anahata chakra which corresponds to the heart, which, surprising enough, has a much stronger magnetic field. Physically the gene is merely a collection of proteins, how to control the DNA depends on the kind of information transmitted on the morphogenetic field.

With the advancement of quantum physics it has been established that everything in our universe is vibrating energy in a state of potential, and all humans, animals, are unique living systems with a unique energy field. Our bodies are connected to the external energy fields.

William A Tiller, Ph.D. of Stanford University states that every substance and organism radiates and absorbs energy via a unique wave field, which then exhibits certain geometrical frequency and radiation characteristics.

The life force gives immediate signals about our energy fields' disturbance, e.g. through the various symptoms through our bodily systems, i.e., pulse, face, meridians, iris, aura, etc. Unless it is understood and responded, they appear in our physical bodies after some time and cause ailments.

When our energy field is in balance and clear and flowing in a healthy pattern, we feel healthy and energetic. The blockages in our energy field are caused by unhealthy life styles, stress, drugs, negative thoughts, mental and emotional disturbances, etc. An unhealthy living or working environment or unhappy marital relationship can prevent the flow of energy too. It is opined that negative planetary positions within our astrological birth charts can cause negative influences on our energy field as well as in our health. Studies have proved that astrological planetary positions are linked between the date of birth (or the date of conception) and a great variety of human health conditions, such as, diseases, abnormalities, personality traits, as well as states of health. Professor Janet Currie and Dr. Hannes Schwandt from Princeton University reported in the Proceedings of the National Academy of Sciences, adds to growing evidence that the timing of pregnancy can influence the health of the baby.

Current scientific experiments have confirmed that living things are connected with the world's energy field. NASA researchers developed a method of detection to measure the living being's energy and information fields, and their errors.

In addition to the bio-resonance testing equipment called NLP panel has already been used in the diagnostics, it is able to detect, explore and reveal past shocking events in our being's information field back to decades.

According to quantum physics, all energy is matter and all matter is energy and thus substance does not exists in itself as principle at all, because everything in our universe is energy.

Quantum physics recognized that all living things are just energy and its various forms of manifestation which explains the holistic connection between the mind-body-spirit, the trinity of health. In 1970, David Cohen of MIT, using a Squid magnetometer enabled to measure magnetic fields around the head produced by brain activities.

We can measure the energy field created by the brain, using electroencephalography which proves that the brain radiates information energy fields.

The micro-nutrients enriched spagyric medicines when applied therapeutically transmit information of the trace elements and are able to penetrate and correct the energy level in the living organisms. Based on the principle of quantum physics, subtle energy information of spagyric essences influence and harmonize the elemental information levels of the consciousness, emotions, behavior, thoughts, connections, soul and spirit, from DNA to cells, it harmonize our energy fields.

Current scientific research provides explanations for how the remedies act on the body and why they are so effective. The existence of "Water Geometry" as well as water's stability, even after it has been converted into steam, was proven in both Pennsylvania and Berkeley Universities, USA in 1995 and 1996. Following distillation, purification and other productions steps, the plants, minerals and metals are transformed into a spagyric tincture. During the course of the production processes the "life energy" contained within the plant, mineral or metal is released from its attachment to material. This energy is comprised of three different active energies: Sal (salt), Sulfur (sulphur), and Mercurius (mercury). Louis Kervran was able to scientifically prove that, specific enzymes cause the transmutation of certain elements such as potassium, hydrogen, magnesium and oxygen into calcium. In the same manner, sodium and hydrogen are transmuted into magnesium, and sodium and oxygen can change into potassium. This phenomenon, which to a certain extent is a natural "alchemical" process, is known as "Biological Transmutation" or the "Kervran Effect".

Dr. Peter Schleicher, immunologist from Munich opined, that spagyric medicines are "effective in influencing and activating" PNEI regulation mechanisms. Scientific experiments at the Atomic Institute in Vienna showed that different plants contain different radiation patterns. Every plant possesses a quite individual field of radiation: a particular 'energy fingerprint'. In a fraction of a second this radiation power senses the 'information' embedded in our body's immune system, which is directly linked to the hormone system and connected with emotion.

Spagyric medicines can effectively correct the human temperament and its connected information-energy level. Chelation or hunger for micro-nutrients or trace elements hinders the optimization of health because of its regulatory and stimulatory influence on enzyme systems; spagyric medicines retrieve missing mineral's information to restore the mind-body-spirit balance.

Spagyric Medicine trigger at the quantum level, and deliver the correct information to activate self-regulation of bodily systems and mechanisms and enhancing its footprint through deep penetration and regulation of cellular functioning which influence at the deepest informational state, respectively the DNAs and RNAs, the higher states of emotional and physical health, thus, influence limbic activity, then hypothalamus and pituitary gland, and finally the sexual organs and adrenal glands, and provides the basis of self-sustainable health.

According to Dr. Peter Schleicher, all levels of this PNI hierarchy can be given regulatory impulses through the help of high quality spagyric medicines.

Even the so-called spontaneous healing of life-threatening diseases such as cancer almost always corresponds with spiritual and mental processes in which there are major changes in the patient's "inner attitude".

Alchemy holds that all things in the universe are interrelated. The idea that there is a relationship between the microcosm and the macrocosm is part of this. Because of that inter- relationship everything can, to a greater or lesser extent, influence, or be influenced by, every other thing. The second is that of 'living Nature', meaning the idea that Nature is dynamic, multi-level, and multivalent. Everything in Nature is potentially a sign of intuitive perception. The third characteristic pertains to a very precise form of 'imagination' and 'mediation'. All elements in the universe are inter-related by means of things that intrinsically possess a mediating character or by means of things within which a mediating quality is thought to inhere, or which can be imbued with that quality, i.e., by somehow being pressed into the service of performing the function of mediation (e.g., images, mandalas, texts, rituals, etc.). The fourth component is called 'transmutation': a term that is derived from alchemy.

'Transmutation' means metamorphosis, and entails a form of gnosis. Together with the idea of 'transmutation' characterisation of esotericism as "both a way of life and an exercise of vision" raises important theoretical considerations that have a direct bearing on understanding what we are calling 'spiritual alchemy'. The alchemist equalled both the alchemical process and the means of the process; alchemical process was tantamount to both self- knowledge and to the knowledge of the divine and that over the course of the alchemical work, there were radical alterations in the conception and the experience of the subject/object relation, causality, and time, resulting in the transmutation of the alchemist himseif. The successful end to the quest for the Philosopher's Stone, which the alchemists initially regarded as external and 'other' to themselves, was spoken of as a return to the prima materia.

Alchemy or Al Kimya (Arabic), or Khemeia (Egyptian) is a form of ceremonial magic commonly believed to be focused on the Transmutation of base metals into precious metals (e.g.: converting lead to gold). The ultimate goal of the Alchemist is to transform the chaotic primordial First Matter (the Khem) into perfection; a goal that is accomplished through spiritual enlightenment.

According to the Masters, in the Process of Alchemical Spiritual Transformation there are 7 Steps:

It represents a further breaking down of the artificial structures of the self by total immersion in the unconscious, non-rational, feminine or rejected part of our minds. It is for the most part, an unconscious process in which our conscious minds let go of control to allow the surfacing of buried material. It is opening the pathways and generating new energy from the waters held back. Dissolution can be experienced as "flow," the bliss of being well used and actively engaged in creative acts without traditional prejudices, personal hang-ups, or established hierarchy getting in the way.

Inwardly, this represents a further breaking down of the artificial structures of the psyche and a unifying of the different aspects. Traditionally the approach was such that the initiates conscious minds must let go of control, opening the channels or pathways and generating new energy from the waters held back; again potentially a painful process. If the approach involves deeper integration and alliance of the subconscious and even the unconscious to a certain degree then dissolution can be experienced as a flow of bliss. It is not traditional psychological therapy but rather a conscious spiritual process through dissolution one becomes more integrated and able to actively engage in creative acts with less personal or cultural prejudice or limited conditioning entering in to the creative process.

Physiologists maintain dissolution as the awakening of the Kundalini, the opening-up of energy channels in the body to recharge and elevate every single cell. Dissolution takes place in the Genital or Root Chakra and involves the lungs and spleen and proceeds upwards.

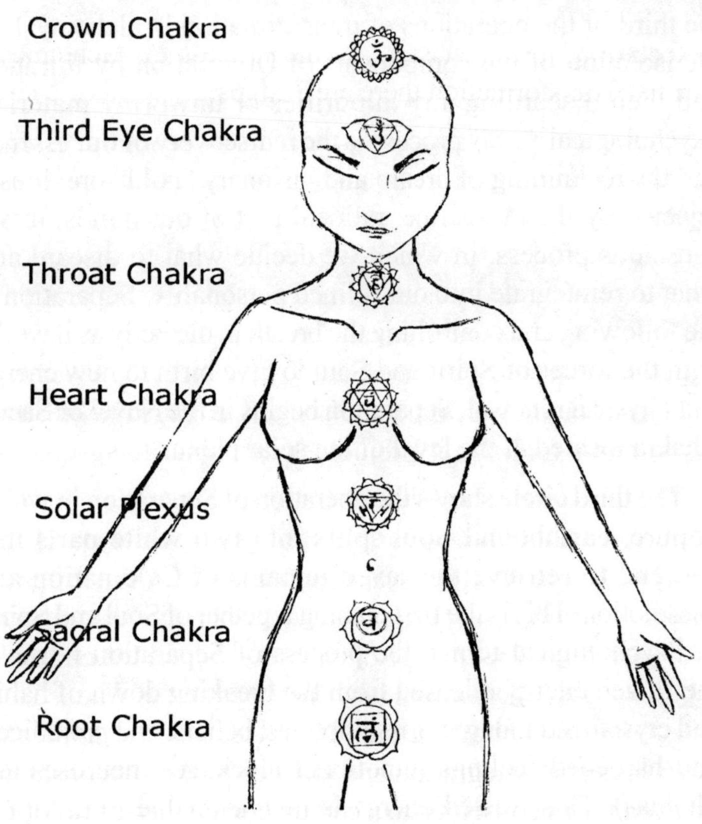

Fig: The Chakra System

The second circle covers Dissolution, it depicts the Soul watching itself undergoing dissolution literally dissolving before it's eyes in the powerful force of the unconscious. It takes the form of dreams, voices, visions and strange feelings which reveal a less ordered and less rational world existing simultaneously with our everyday life, also reflecting back from the pool of dissolution is the white image of the essence of the Soul which is exposed in this operation. Just as Calcination works on the mind and ego to destroy deceptions and impure thoughts, so dissolution work on the heart and release buried emotions that conceal or distort our true nature.

The Third circle covers the process of Separation which is the third of the operations of transformation in alchemy. It is the isolation of the components of Dissolution by filtration and then discarding any impurities or unworthy material. Psychologically, this process is the rediscovery of our essence and the reclaiming of dream and visionary "gold" previously rejected by the masculine, rational part of our minds. It is a conscious process, in which we decide what to discard and what to reintegrate into our refined personality. Separation is the following and controlling the breath in the body as it works with the forces of Spirit and Soul to give birth to new energy and physical renewal. Separation begins in the Naval or Sacral Chakra located at the level of the solar plexus.

The third circle shows the operation of Separation in which impure, earthbound Soul splits into two white parts that descend to retrieve the saved remains of Calcination and Dissolution. This is the first coming together of Soul and Spirit. In Psychological terms, the process of Separation retrieves the frozen energy released from the breaking down of habits and crystalized thoughts (assumptions, beliefs, and prejudices) and hardened feelings (emotional blockages, neuroses and phobias). This wasted energy is now available to drive our Spiritual Transformation. To summarize, Separation is the letting go of the self-inflicted restraints to our true nature and saving the hidden essence, which becomes the subject of the following operations. The essence is made up of the best parts of our Spirit and Soul, our Mind and Heart. Separation delivers the retrieved Spiritual Essence safely through the processes of Calcination and Dissolution to the First Incarnation, which is Earthly Conjunction.

Conjunction or reuniting is the fourth of the seven operations of alchemy. It is the joining together of the saved elements from Separation into a new substance. Psychologically, It is empowerment of our true selves, the union of both the feminine and masculine sides of our personalities into a new belief system or an intuitive state of consciousness. The integration of the conscious and unconscious aspects of the Psyche, which, the alchemist referred to it as the Philosopher's Stone, and after it is achieved, the adept is able to clearly discern what needs to be done to achieve lasting enlightenment. In other words, this corresponds to the union of both the masculine and feminine sides of our nature into a unified state of consciousness. With this unification comes the potential for direct non-linear knowing that is more than intuition; but rather a direct knowing by being able align with the cosmic mind. Physiologically, Conjunction is using the bodies sexual energies for personal transformation which takes place in the body at the level of the Heart Chakra.

The fourth circle depicts the Quintessence recovered from the preceding operations on the realm of the psychic mind. On the personal level, the union of both masculine and feminine sides of our personalities into a new belief system that must still be nurtured to survive. The Child of the Philosophers, in a realm of Consciousness grows in strength to achieve lasting enlightenment.

Fermentation is the Fifth cycle in the Alchemy of Transformation. It is the chemical breakdown of a substance by bacteria, yeasts, or other micro-organisms, especially that which is involved in the making of beers, wines, and spirits in which sugar is converted to ethyl alcohol. Fermentation is a two-stepped process that begins with the decomposition of the psychic resulting in the death and spiritual rebirth to a new level of being. The Fermentation phase then begins with the introduction of new life into the product of conjunction to strengthen it and habituate its survival.

Fermentation is the growth of a Ferment (bacteria) in organic solutions, which occurs in the fermenting of grapes to produce wine. The process starts with the inspiration of spiritual power from above that reanimates, energizes, and enlightens the alchemist. Out of the remains of his waste psyche comes the yellow ferment, which appears like a golden wax flowing out of the fowl matter of the Soul. Its arrival is announced by a brilliant display of colors and meaningful visions called the "Peacock's Tail." Fermentation can be achieved through various practices that include intense prayer, desire for mystical union, melting down of the personality, regression therapy, religious practices and meditation.

It is the rousing of Kundalini energy to heal, sustain and enlighten to a new level of being. It is expressed as vibratory tones and spoken truths emerging from the Throat Chakra.

Distillation is the Sixth cycle in the Transformation, which literally means to purify a liquid by heating it until it vaporizes, then cooling and condensing the vapor and collecting the resulting liquid, often with a solvent. It is the boiling and condensation of the fermented solution to increase its purity, which takes place in the distilling of wine to make brandy. Psychologically, the agitation and sublimation of psychic forces is necessary to ensure that no impurities from the ego or personality are incorporated into the next and final process. The alchemist thought of this phase as working with the heavenly element Mercury to extract, thrift and rebuilt the metals. The ferment, the soft amalgam or balsam resulting from this operation, must be hardened into a Stone before it can be made permanent, and the final phase of distillation is a sublimation in which the vapor turns solid, or the Spirit is made perceptive.

Alchemists opine that distillation consists of a variety of introspection techniques that raise the content of the psyche to the highest level possible. Free from personality, ego and emotions. Distillation is raising the self from the lower regions of the body to the brain (western alchemists call it the circulation of light and eastern alchemists or siddhas call it attainment of siddhi), where it eventually becomes a wondrous solidifying light full of power. Distillation is often compared to the culmination in the Third Eye, at the level of the pituitary and pineal glands, in between the brows or Ajna or Third Eye Chakra.

The important Distillation process is referred to in the Emerald Tablet "It rises from Earth to Heaven, and then descends again to the Earth, and receives Power from Above and from Below." It is the transformational stage where we spiritually and emotionally attain maturity to merge with the collective conscious and unconscious or the microcosm. The reason one can maintain his/ her balance after having arrived at the distillation stage is that neither the ego nor the personality could take over the purified soul and hence one can therefore feel oneness with the universal spirit without any seizing or intrusion.

Distillation makes us pure and balanced in serenely powerful ways. A distilled person would surrender to the cosmic forces while celebrating and honoring the existence of the lower ones.

Coagulation is the seventh and final cycle in the Psychological Transformation or Mystical and Spiritual Alchemy rather than the Physical Transmutation of base metals into Gold. The Process of Transformation is seen to be one of a series of seven stages of attaining the higher personality from the lower personality. It is the precipitation or sublimation of the purified ferment from Distillation.

Coagulation incarnates and releases the Ultima Materia of the Soul, the Astral Body, which the alchemists also referred to as the Greater or Philospher's Stone. Using the magical Stone, the alchemists believed they could exist on all levels of reality. Physiologically, this stage is marked by the release of the Elixir in the blood that rejuvenates the body into a perfect vessel of health. In the brain a necter is said to be released through the interaction of light from the phallic-shaped pineal gland and matter from the vulva of the pituitary. This heavenly food or viaticum both nourishes and energizes the cells without any waste products being produced. These physiological and psychological processes create a beam of solid light that emerges through the Crown or Gold Chakra.

The Great Work of alchemy consists of stabilizing this vision of Light into a full realization. The by-product is that the body-building power of the subconscious changes the alchemist him/herself into a new creature.

The oldest source book of knowledge on the planet is the Rig Veda. The word Soma means "to extract" or "press out" hence the association with elixir. Within the Rig Veda is the Ninth Mandala, an entire book devoted to Soma praising it as an elixir of enlightenment. The secret of Soma and its preparation, as well as the secret distillation of the Vedas themselves, was called the Madhuvidya or the Honey Doctrine.

There has been much debate over the years as to the definition and identity of Soma since it is veiled in symbolism and metaphor in the Vedas. Internally, Soma is associated with the pin point of transcendence located in the head center. The symbolism of the pinpoint (center of a circle) and Soma are both associated with the Moon. The pin point and crescent Moon are seen at the top of the Sanskrit Om symbol of infinity.

Through advanced meditation, Soma nectar is said to drop from the point down to the Throat or Vishuddhi Chakra where one drinks the internal nectar. The symbolism of Soma is also associated with the Fountain of Life, Dew of Heaven, and Lord Shiva. Somasundara is another name for Shiva. The complete union of Kundalini Shakti with Soma Shiva results in Samadhi or self realization.

"Thus you will have the Glory of the Whole World. All obscurity will be clear to you. This is the Strong Power of All Powers because it Overcomes Everything Fine and Penetrates Everything Solid."—the Emerald Tablet.

The transformation process is the "Journey into Self", or Union with the Higher Self," and is called by Dr. Carl G. Jung "The Process of Individuation."

The alchemical principal of "solve et coagula," or dissolve and coagulate, has been used at each stage of the process. In other words, the form the soul is caught in at the time (the self) must first be dissolved in order to free the soul so that it can rise (in consciousness) to experience a purer and subtler form, which can then be re-coagulated and experienced as the "new self." However, in stage four as the soul incarnates, or descends into the worldly body, the latter has been tempered to be a more suitable vehicle or psyche, which is then coagulated with the soul to form the "self" that has awakened the body and mind to express its nature (the spirit has been materialised and the material body spiritualised). The contribution of Alchemy to modern Psychotherapy, modern studies of Alchemy, the most notable being Jung's "Psychology and Alchemy", have changed our understanding and interpretation of dreams. In 1946 his work on the "Psychology of the Transference Interpreted in Conjunction with a set of Alchemical Illustrations" revealed a very different light on transference in psychotherapy, which until the time of this publication was influenced mainly by the writings of Sigmund

Freud, i.e. that transference was simply a phenomenon that reflected the influence of the parent-child relationship. Jung's work on alchemy showed instead that the transference dreams and experiences of his clients were principally concerned with an inner process of individuation. This process does of course acknowledge the importance of the experience of bonding with and separating from the parental figures, but it also goes way beyond this by envisaging life as a continual process of development. Thus the projections of the clients onto the therapist reflect something of their own inner psychic world rather than Freud's view that the client was basically experiencing the therapist as a parent figure. The greatest contribution that alchemy makes to psychotherapy is its understanding of the process of transformation. It is applicable on the one hand to the simple process of undergoing a change in the way we see the world and at the other end of the scale it provides vital background knowledge to the understanding of the process of spiritual transformation. Jung's texts "Alchemical Studies" (1931-54) and "Mysterium Coniunctionis" (1956) are classical studies on the subject of Symbolism and Alchemical Process of Transformation.

Alchemy is the study of the forces of creation in the macrocosm of the universe. Once these principles are mastered, the individual (or microcosm) can utilize these same forces to trans-form and enhance his or her own life. When practiced on the higher spiritual level, alchemy is a powerful force for the evolution of soul, which is the expression of the First Matter in us. By working in the inner laboratory of the mind, initiates learn alchemistic meditation and work with the Three Essentials to achieve actual transmutation.

Dennis Hauck has noted that lasting transformation takes place where the work is accomplished on all levels of reality. "The material, the spiritual, and the physical" and these levels are all mysteriously inter-related in the subtle essence of Kundalini awakening.

13

Sexual Alchemy

"In the beginning God created the heaven and the earth. "And the earth was without form, and void; and darkness was upon the face of the deep. And the Spirit of God moved upon the face of the waters.

"And God said, Let there be light: and there was light,

"And God saw the light, that it was good: and God divided the light from the darkness,

"And God called the light Day, and the darkness he called Night And the evening and the morning were the first day.

"And God said, Let there be a firmament in the midst of the waters, and let it divide the waters from the waters.

"And God made the firmament, and divided the waters that were under the firmament from the waters that were above the firmament: and it was so.

"And God called the firmament Heaven, And the evening and the morning were the second day.

"And God said, Let the waters under the heaven be gathered together unto one place, and let the dry land appeal': and it was so. And God called the dry land Earth,' and the gathering together of the waters called he Seas: and God saw that it was good."——Holy Bible, Genesis 1:1

If a human being wishes to create his bodies of liberation, in order to self-realize as a Master of the Universe he must then create as God did, by fertilizing his seminal system in order for the interior universe to emerge from it.

The sprout is the semen, if we wish to create as the Gods, we must fertilize the Sprout with the vivifying fire in order for our bodies of perfection, with which we realize ourselves as Masters of the Universe, to emerge from it.

Sprout is a mixture of water and fire, The water of the Sprout is the receptacle of the fire, The earth is reduced to water, and the water is the receptacle of the fire. Our material body, which is our individual earth, is reduced to the water of the semen. Thus, if we fertilize the Sprouts of the semen with the fire of the Spirit, the Child of Gold of Sexual Alchemy emerges. Hence, if we wish to create our interior universe, we must create as God did when He created the universe.

It is necessary to divide the waters from the waters in order to place these (the waters) above, in our Divine Heaven (firmament), where the glory of the Innermost (Spirit) shines. This is achieved by placing what is material and crude into the profundity of the Abyss, and by raising our life force by sublimating our seminal energy. This is a work of Sexual Alchemy.

"Separate that Spirituous earth from the dense or crude by means of a gentle heat, with much attention. In great measure it ascends from the earth up to heaven, and descends".

—Hennes Trismegistus

The eternal essence of the Universe resides here in our seminal system. If God had to fertilize the waters of the eternal essence with the fire in order to create the Universe, we must do the same by fertilizing the waters of our eternal essence, which is our semen, with the fire of the Kundalini. This is done in order to make our interior Universe emerge and to convert ourselves into ineffable Gods. This is known as Sexual Alchemy. The supra-celestial waters of the Sprouts are pure semen, and from this semen the Universe emerged.

This supra-celestial water of creation is a very pure, flexible and inflamed substance, but it never consumes itself. This is the Paradise where Adam lived before the downfall. Let us fertilize the semen. Let us divide the waters from the waters, by placing what is material and crude into the Abyss and by placing the divine and sublime within our interior firmament, This is how we can convert ourselves into Gods of the Universe. Our seminal system, our earth, is now void and entirely without form, The darkness is now upon the face of the Abyss and the Spirit of God is moving upon the face of our seminal waters.

Let us create light, let us create it by extracting the light from the darkness by means of Sexual Alchemy.

The light is good; let us depart ourselves from the darkness. Let us divide the waters from the waters, in other words, the light from the darkness, and let us gather the tenebrous waters in the Abyss in order to discover the dry matter, which is a rich interior Universe, the bodies of perfection. Thus, we self-realize as Masters of the interior and the delicate Eden, where the lights of the heaven shine and from where every living creature emerges.

The human mechanism is a composite of the physical body an accumulation of food consumed; the mental body the intellect and memory part that makes individuals function in specific ways; and the energy body the fundamental upon which these two are housed. What is beyond this is non-physical.

The compulsive and cyclical nature of the body and mind render themselves a barrier for higher possibilities. Sexual Alchemy is to go beyond, so that compulsiveness of the body and mind does not keep us trapped in our limitations. It is about learning to use the body, not as oneself, but as a stepping-stone to deliver this being to the highest possible dimension.

Sexual Alchemy is not about uninhibited sexuality, as assumed by many. Sexuality is a fundamental instinct instilled in our bodies to ensure the species perpetuates itself. This is a basic requirement. At the same time, one must know the limitations beyond which it will not carry us. It is only on recognising the limitations and the longing to touch other dimensions enters, that Sexual Alchemy become relevant.

In Sexual Alchemy, it is not that someone is using just sexuality to grow. They are using every aspect to grow. Sexual needs can be fulfilled by forming relationships for that purpose. Using spiritual process to fulfill sexual compulsions is reprehensible and irresponsible. It can lead to various levels of loss because the tantric process is not only used for the individual's spiritual growth, but also to create an energetic space to support other possibilities that bring well-being to many.

The simple principle of Sexual Alchemy is, whatever can take you down can also take you up. The ways in which a man usually sinks in his life are through food, alcoholic drink and sexuality. Sexual Alchemy uses the same three vehicles to rise up. Unlike sexuality, which tends to find release at the lower level of the energy system, Sexual Alchemy is about building our energies to the fountain-head of the uppermost dimension of the energy system, so that one's energies spill from the top. Of the different energy manifestations in the body referred to as the chakras spilling from the top three is considered the highest. If you have to build up to this, every basic instinct, including the sexual instinct, emotions, intellect and survival process must be used to build and hype the energy system. The intention is to deploy all instincts for which a certain amount of energy is dedicated in the body. If one goes into an actual sexual act, the build-up and the purpose of it will be lost.

Philosophically, Sexual Alchemy means you are able to use your energies to make things happen. If you can make your mind razor sharp to cut through everything, this is also one kind of tantra. If you make your energies work upon your heart to become utterly loving and you can burst forth with enormous love that just overwhelms everyone, this is also Sexual Alchemy. If you make your physical body enormously powerful to make it do incredible feats, this is also Sexual Alchemy. Or if you can make your energies do things by itself without employing the body, mind or emotion, this is also Sexual Alchemy.

Intimacy is generally understood only as two bodies touching. The body is not intimate enough for one who is on the spiritual path. The physical body is an accumulation from outside, so in the tantric and yogic systems, the body is never considered an intimate part of you. Only when the subtle energies meet and mingle and a Spiritual Teacher's energies overwhelm and override the disciple's energies, it leads to an orgasmic experience: a union, but not of the sexual kind.

There seems a metaphysical or symbolic correspondence between the planetary and metallurgical attributions of sexual alchemy and the chakras. The qualities of the metals correspond to the planets and chakras as follows:

Lead	Saturn	Sacral Plexus
Iron	Mars	Sexual Ganglion
Tin	Jupiter	Solar Plexus
Gold	Sun	Cardiac Plexus
Copper	Venus	Pharyngeal Plexus
Silver	Moon	Pituitary Body
Quicksilver	Mercury	Pineal Gland

Lead being the Earth, Mercury being the Holy Spirit which travels between Earth and the center of the Universe and Sulphur being the Sun or the Central Spiritual Sun. These three comprise the Holy Trinity and are talked about in the Guided meditation described in the Emerald Tablet of Hermes Trismegistus. This Guided meditation is the same as the Kundalili Tantra both Microcosmic and Macrocosmic.

As with Gurdjieff and his Reciprocal maintenance the movement of the Energies from Heaven to Earth between the Father and the Son, between the central Spiritual Sun and the Earth has the effect of transmuting Energy Blockages which always are trying to stop this flow of energy.

These Alchemical meditations are in order to Transmute base metal, lead, the Energy Blockages in the Earth and in human beings into Spiritual Gold, The Earth being transmuted into a Sacred Planet and the Human Being, filled with evil blockages, into An Enlightened Being and Ascended master.

Thus, Energy Enhancement teaches the Real Spiritual Alchemy Gaining Spiritual Energy and purifying the body from its Energy Blockages.

Sexual Alchemy is not concerned exclusively with consciousness, but also seeks the subtle transformation of the body, so that the physical level is also brought into perfect equilibrium. Thus, the alchemical metals may be considered analogous to the chakras of the practitioners. We can draw another parallel among the three major principles of alchemy and those of Hindu Philosophy, which are known as the qualities.

Mercury.......Sattva

Sulphur.........Rajas

Salt..............Tamas

The quality of Mercury is vital and reflective; it equates with the spiritual principles of goodness and intelligence; Sattva guna (characteristic) is illuminative. The quality of Sulphur is fiery and passionate like the principles of Rajas, which incites desire, attachment and action. The quality of Salt is arrestive and binding, and reflects the gross inertia of matter, which is much like Tamas. These gunas and the three alchemical substances symbolize spirit, soul and body. Another "alchemical" way the gunas were applied concerns food: sattvic foods incline one toward meditation and the spiritual life (fruits, vegetables, nuts, and grains); rajasic food (spicy rich food) are stimulating ; tamasic food (animal flesh) incites the basic instincts.

The concept of four basic elements, harmonized in a fifth, is also common to both alchemy and yoga doctrines. The Indian elements are known as Tattvas. They are: Akasha (quintessence); Tejas or Agni (fire); Apas (water); Vayu (air); Prithivi (earth). Furthermore, the preparation for the practice of both alchemy and yoga requires a moral or ethical preparation. Both stress that evil tendencies should be overcome while positive virtues are developed. This includes both behavior and the purification of various body centers. The objective is not wealth, but health or wholeness.

Sexual Alchemy also speaks of a "secret fire", which is often compared to a serpent or dragon. Here again, we find the correspondence to Kundalini, the serpent-power. Alchemy is performed by the aid of Mercury, the illuminative principle, and the powers of the sun and moon. Sexual Alchemy works in three channels in the subtle body. One equates with the sun, another with the moon. They are called ida and pingala. The third, or harmonizing channel, is known as sushumna, and is associated with illumination. The twin serpents twine together and open the third way, as shown in the Cadeusus.

Sexual Alchemy literally means "woven together". The central theme of Alchemy is a cosmic feminine force who, under the form of a goddess, is the incarnation of the feminine aspects of every divinity. This feminine energy is also known as the counterpart of a cosmic masculine force. This feminine force often adopts beneficial forms helping the adepts attain perfect union with Absolute. Sexual Alchemy contains five themes :

1. the creation of the world.
2. the destruction or dissolution of the world
3. the ways one can intensely worship the Almighty in all his feminine and masculine aspects, or, in other words, the ineffable fusion with one of the countless masculine and feminine divinities.
4. the obtaining of the paranormal powers (Siddhi).
5. various ways and methods to achieve an intimate and ineffable fusion with the Supreme Being, in meditation. Often Sexual Alchemy is synonymous to Kundalini Yoga. The Alchemical texts are generally presented under the form of a dialog between the cosmic feminine and masculine forces. They present ways to accelerate the spiritual progress and then to attain the divine perfection by the awakening and perfect control of the cosmic energy Kundalini which is asleep at the base of the spine, in root chakra. Through a vast series of physical and mental techniques that have very positive effects over the health and wellbeing, the control of energies, the profound harmonization of emotions, the discipline and focalization of the mind could be achieved. It also uses sacred geometrical paintings (Yantra or Talisman) and sacred words (Mantra) which are tools for entering in a process of Resonance with the beneficial forces of the Macrocosm. In certain practices, sexual continence allows for the Transmutation and Sublimation of the huge sexual potential, producing a rapid and

beneficial transformation of the human being. All these processes can be achieved either by being sexually abstinent in conjunction with the tantra yoga techniques or by being sexually continent, and over time, they produce a gradual elevation of the consciousness until it reaches the state of Ananda (Ecstasy or Eternal bliss).

This mode of thought is associated with the left hemisphere of the human brain and generally takes the form of a subvocal monologue or dialogue. It is only this sort of thinking that mysticism rejects.

At the same time that one stops verbal thinking in mystical sex, one is completely aware of what is going on. Mysticism recommends that one fully, totally, directly experience and participate actively and creatively during lovemaking. One is completely awake, aware, involved and absorbed , but without describing every part of the experience to oneself in words as it's going on.

In mystical intercourse, lovers are more mentally aware, able to concentrate and get into it, by virtue of the fact that they are not thinking, because the direct perception of whatever is happening is no longer filtered by what we usually call the rational mind.

Mystical intercourse favors the creative, perceptive, intuitive, feeling of experiencing directly. Without describing every sensation to oneself, without thinking, one just feels the physical sensations that occur.

In conclusion, during mystical lovemaking men and women are open to sensation, perceiving it without evaluating it.

In Western culture, Sexual Alchemy or Tantra Yoga is being described in such a way that it is supposed to mean uninhibited sex. It has been willfully misinterpreted. This is because books on tantra have been written by people who just want to sell books. They have never encountered real spiritual practitioners of the East and do not know real Tantra in any way.

The word "tantra" literally means a sacred methodology to achieve the union with the supreme power. This is an inner technology. These are subjective methods not objective methods. Sex is related to release of body fluids in genitals whereas Sexual Alchemy or Tantra Yoga is related to releasing sacred nectar in Sahasrara Chakra by awakning Kundalini. Contrary to the aberrations proliferated by the malevolent, Alchemy or Tantra is life lived with intensity, in a superior way.

Sexual Alchemy seeks to arouse the latent power of the Kundalini serpent so it rises up the Chakra centers until it opens the third eye of mystical vision and illumination. Alchemists apply slow heat to their alchemical vessel to sublimate and refine the contents therein.

"*Syzygy or conjunction of the macrocosmic Unity with the microcosmic triunity. The entire process of the elaboration of the Philosopher's Stone is symbolized here ...* "

——Stanislas Klassowski de Rolla

Alchemists perform transmutation in two ways;

1) to recognize what goes on in his body, and
2) to use this knowledge to control subconscious processes by awakening self-consciousness so that his/her physical processes has no influence on increased vitality. This supercharge of libido then awakens the spiritual vision of the pineal gland to full activity. So, let us perform transformation within ourselves, by means of Sexual Alchemy.

The Alchemical Gold of Sexual Alchemy:

"Alchemy is the art of liberating parts of the Cosmos from temporal existence and achieving perfection which, for metals is gold, and for man, longevity, then immortality and, finally, redemption. Material perfection was sought through the action of a preparation (Philosopher's Stone for metals; Elixir of

Life for humans), while spiritual ennoblement resulted from some form of inner revelation or other enlightenment"

-H.J.Sheppard (1986: 13-17)

In the laboratories, there were apparatus of different shapes and materials, needed to maintain Alchemical operations as combination, heating, evaporation, separation and dissolution. At the spiritual and mystical level, the human body was a furnace to the human soul and mind in the process of transmutation.

In Western and Eastern alchemical texts, the sexual discharge of the woman is referred to as the Red Lion (Sulphur), and the ejaculate (Salt) as the White Eagle.

The Elixir is the conjunction of the fluids produced by the union of the male and the female, and is symbolized by Mercury.

In an ancient alchemical treatise called "The Sounding of the Trumpet," it is written: "In the Lunar Stone is the white sulphur, in the Solar Stone red sulphur, and the Mercurial Stone embraces both, which is the strength of the whole Magistery." This alludes to the exchange of fluids, one into the other vessel.

Red is the color of youth on the Tree of Life and has become known to most by its association with the Phallus, Mars (the God of War), and the Kundalini. Red, is also the heraldic substitute for the metal Gold, a metal usually attributed to the Sun and possessing male qualities. At first glance it is easy to perceive this as conflict in archetypes, the female quality in youth is a higher expression of the passionate qualities expressed in the root of Fire and unbridled passion. Youth also represents the destruction of the old so that something new can exist, and this will remind those of us that understand a woman's cycle of the regeneration of the surface of the uterus which occurs during menstruation.

The physical manifestation of the Elixir of Life, Alchemical Gold, or the Stone of The Philosophers is symbolized by the Four Elements: Fire, Wind, Water and Earth, the Garden of Eden, whose magical image is that of a beautiful young maiden sitting upon a cube holding an apple between her legs.

The essence of any individual is bisexual in nature, we bear both male and female qualities. The contrast in the behavior of men and women is mainly due to our physical and emotional embodiments.

The idea behind sexual alchemy is that the 'Qi' or 'Prana' must be brought to balance through the union of its opposite represented by the male and female counterpart. Once this is done the "Qi" will experience total freedom of expression which will rise above the confines of the human body and social conditioning. Once this occurs, Union with God is possible.

The idea of "Alchemical Gold", as it pertains to the Elixir which is said useful to delay the effects of aging, prolong life, and healing illness comes from the fact mentioned above: that the human body uses the finest nutrients for the development of masculine and feminine secretions. Once the practice of absorbing these fluids is repeated over many years, the ultimate result will be secretions of the highest purity, their potency being greatly increased each time, until the consummation of such secretions has the potential to heal all the diseases. This is called the fruit of liberation; the "Alchemical Gold".

14

Spagyric Meditation

Expansion Stage

Lie on a bed or on the floor for minimum 10 minutes. Close your eyes, and visualize firmly and clearly the "growth" of your energetic body. Make it grow more and more, perceiving the cosmic beneficial energy that allows its growth.

Continue to expand your aura until you have reached the ceiling of your room, or the sky above, in case you are outdoors.

Get used to this sensation gradually, performing this exercise for two-three days in a row before clearly and definitely begin to notice its effects: a vitalizing, euphoric sensation, as well as a state of inner peace.

Further on, visualize your aura growing even more, beyond the room. Thus your aura may become as large as the place you live in. Expand your aura even more, as much as you can.

The limits do not exist. You may even feel your aura is as big as your town or the whole planet or even the solar system. Expand your aura until you feel you have the whole universe inside of you.

Perform this expansion technique for seven days, and then repeat it reversed (contraction) for another seven days.

Contraction Stage

Lie in bed or on the floor, just as mentioned before. Perceive your body and then begin the contraction stage as follows:

Imagine your body becoming small, until it is the size of an atom, and furthermore, until this atom ends up dissolving into something unique and eternal that resides within you.

At the end of the seven days of practicing this technique, you will realize that you can become so small from a subtle point of view, that you almost cannot "locate" yourselves.

Through this experiences, you will realize as well that through the expansion stage you can become as infinite as the universe, and through the contraction you cam become as small and invisible as an atom.

Therefore, perform these exercises for seven days in a row, just as described above.

Among the beneficial effects you will notice in just ten-fifteen minutes of daily practice for two weeks are: state of inner harmony, plenitude and happiness, balance, and in the advanced stages, the practitioner may even attain Samadhi.

The Secret to Successful Meditation

Many of us have noticed that when we try to focus on a certain issue, subject or phenomenon, most often our mind would not stay with us, wandering about to things we sometimes barely become aware of.

However, do not despair, as an adequate mental practice may solve this problem.

Focus is a special, disciplined form of attention, which implies a contraction in the field of attention, so that there is no interference of the irrelevant stimuli, which usually distract us. Our whole consciousness is now directed in one direction only, or in other words we are focused.

The benefits of a great power of concentration in the daily life are obvious:

You will be able to perform your duties more rapidly and effectively, and also to keep in mind more details associated to them. Most of the mistakes people usually do are caused by the lack of attention while performing a particular action.

Through practice you may train your mind to be more clear and insightful, regardless of the action itself. Thus you create the conditions for the mind to go back inwards, to the true source of existence, the divine Self or Macrocosm .

You can learn to focus through practice, just as any other thing. Just as focusing is essential in meditation, training your attention to concentrate on one object only is the optimal way to attain great concentration.

Enhance the Capacity to focus

Take a common word, for instance "Light" or "Air". Write it down on a piece of paper and then write the first word associated to the one you chose and that is associated to it.

Come back to your first choice and write down another word related to the first, return to the first one and so on, until you run out of related words.

After this, stick with the initial word, keep it in mind, and focus on it, without thinking about it. Continue the exercise for at least 15 minutes once a day, for a month in a row. By the end of the month, you will surely notice a greater capacity of mental focus.

Focus on Breathing

1. The first essential step in the practice of meditation is concentration. The mind has to have an object to focus upon.

Whenever your mind "runs" away from the object you chose to meditate upon (be it because of boredom, unwanted thoughts, or tiredness) you have to bring it back gently, but firmly.

You can meditate on absolutely anything. Nonetheless, especially in the early stages of meditation it is recommended that you chose a simple and/or rhythmical object of meditation.

Such an object is your breath. The breath is simple, and rhythmical, permanently getting out and then in, up and down, flux and reflux.

Moreover, the breath cannot be associated to a particular person or characteristic. It is the sustainer of life, vital to our existence, and still people have become so accustomed to it, they hardly pay any attention.

2. Find a quiet place and stay there, either in an asana or posture or on a chair, important is to have your spine straight and the head on the same line with the spine.

   Focus on your breath and keep this concentration steady, without any interruptions for as long as you can, refusing to let yourself be distracted by any thoughts or exterior events.

   Perceive the air you inhale, the short break between inhalation and exhalation, the air you exhale, and the short following break – this time between inhalation and exhalation.

   Do not intervene in the natural rhythm of the breath, let it flow by itself, and notice how it becomes more and more tranquil as your body and mind relax in meditation.

   If you are beginners in the practice of mind focus, make the session last 5-10 minutes. Try to make the sessions daily and at the same time. After several weeks of practice, extend the time allocated to this issue to 15-20 minutes.

   However, do not push things too much before their time. Meditation is not about forcing yourself, it is about being at peace with yourself and although it has certain connections to a kind of rigor, it has more to do with flexibility than rigidity.

   It is also important that you realize that until you reach a certain degree of mastery in spagyric meditation, thoughts and emotions out of control will cross your meditation.

   Do not be frustrated and do not pay much attention. Let them go through you, without allowing them to disturb your inner peace and focus. Do not fight them in an attempt of casting them away, but let them move through you.

Regardless of their apparent importance, do not hang up on them, and do not allow them to “flow” from one into another, distracting you in this manner.

Nonetheless, even when you realize you have been distracted, return to your meditation firmly, but gently. This gentleness is important, as your mind will never obey any “harsh” command, but will always go with the flow of a gentle direction.

Pay attention to your breath, be patient and avoid negative thinking. A wandering mind only proves an acute need for meditation, so that it finally calms down.

It is an indication of how little control you have over your mind at this point.

The key is the gratitude for that part of your consciousness that has signaled your distraction and that made it possible for you to return to your meditation.

15

Hermetic Philosophy

Hippocrates, the father of modern medicine, nearly 2,500 years ago observed a connection between the movements of the stars and disease, writing that "the contribution of astronomy to medicine is not a small one but a very great one indeed." Doctors of the time believed the movements of the celestial bodies, which were used for marking the passage of time, had a powerful influence on one's health.

Franz Anton Mesmer in his 1766 thesis submitted to Vienna University established the influence of the planets on the human body, in which he first publicly presented his account of the harmonic forces at work in the microcosm.

> *"The world is the Macrocosm and man the Microcosm, and the elements of all that exists in the former exist in the latter. All the influences that come from the sun, the planets, the stars, act therefore invisibly upon man, and if these influences are evil they will produce evil effects."*

> *"An evil astral influence does not poison the whole world, but only those places where causes for infection exist. If no germs of disease exist in our atmosphere, the astral influences coming from the outside will cause no harm. if evil elements exist in the sphere of our soul, they attract such astral influences as may develop diseases."*

> *"The moon exercises a very bad influence, especially at the time of the new moon, which may be very injurious*

for persons whose sidereal bodies possess magnetic elements that will attract that influence, and the conjunction of the moon with certain other planets may make her influence still more injurious. For instance, a conjunction of the Moon, Venus, and Mars may give rise to the plague; a conjunction with Saturn, to certain acute diseases, etc., but no evil influence can develop a disease where the germ of that disease does not already exist."

"The seat of the Sun in the microcosm is in the heart, that of the moon is in the brain. The Moon's influence is cold; and insane people have been called "lunatics" because they are often injuriously affected by the Moon, whose influence acts upon the brain and stimulates the sexual passions, and causes injurious dream and hallucinations."

"Every organ in the human body is formed by the action of certain principles that exist in the Universe, and the former attract the corresponding activity in the latter. Thus the heart is in sympathy with the elements of the sun, the brain with the moon, the gall-bladder with Mars, the kidneys with Venus, the lungs with Mercury, the liver with Jupiter, the spleen with Saturn, etc. There are many stars in the great firmament of the Universe, and there are many germs hidden in the little world of Man, and the high influences the low; and in the Macrocosm and microcosm all things stand in intimate sympathetic relationship with each other, for all are the children of one universal father."

"Good or evil influence comes down from the Sun, the Moon, or the stars; the action of the macrocosmic influences stimulates the corresponding elements (Corpora Microcosmic Astralia) existing in man into action. The same element which produces Mars, Venus

or Jupiter in the sky, exists also in the body of man; because the latter is the son of the astral body of the macrocosm in the same sense as the physical body of man is a son of the earth."

"To be a physician, it is not sufficient to know the anatomy of the physical body, you should also know that of the astral body, you show know not merely a part, but the whole constitution of the macrocosm and the microcosm of man." - Paracelsus

Frater Albertus teaches five laws of Astrology, of these, the fourth law is the major key, the Law of the Four Elements.

The Fire triangle links Aries, Leo and Sagittarius The Earth triangle links Taurus, Virgo and Capricorn The Air triangle links Gemini, Libra and Aquarius and The Water triangle links Cancer, Scorpio and Pisces.

The Planets; Sun, Moon, Mercury, Venus and Mars symbolises the urges which are ego-oriented and are readily available to consciousness.

The Sun is the heart of the solar system, and the most important symbol in the birth chart. It symbolises the individual's urge to become himself. It is the urge for self-awareness and wholeness. The Sun sign in a birth chart is not a set of pre-existent and crystallized behaviour patterns, but rather it indicates those qualities which the individual can potentially make conscious. In fact, it is his task to make these qualities conscious through the channel of his unique individuality. For example, the Sun in Aries does not make a man headstrong and impulsive, "but it suggests that he needs to cultivate a sense of the vitality of life, an ability to assert himself in the outside world, a capacity to initiate change and meet challenges creatively, if he is to become whole."

The Sun is a positive or masculine "planet" because it is associated with that side of life which concerns will, consciousness, decision, and impact on the environment in other words, an active principle. It is more "accessible" to men than to women, because it reflects an easier impulse for a man to make conscious.

The Moon symbolises the urge towards unconsciousness, the past, and immersion in the flow of feeling of the mass currents of life, without the struggle required for self-consciousness. The Moon is a symbol of the mother, both personal and archetypal, and the womb. It is the urge to satisfy emotional needs through relationship and the merging of identity. It symbolises the instinctual or non-rational nature.

The Moon also suggests, by its placement in the birth chart, "that sphere of life wherein the individual seeks a symbolic sleep, an unconsciousness, an escape or refuge" - where his needs will dominate rather than his will.

In general, the Sun is a symbol of consciousness and the Moon of the unconscious in a man's horoscope; and in a woman's the Moon symbolises consciousness and the Sun the unconscious. The Sun and Moon are two halves of the same unity. It is their harmonious integration which is the true sacred marriage, the inner union.

Mercury is not merely a symbol of the intellect, but rather symbolises the way we perceive and order our perceptions so that they can be comprehended and communicated. Which is primarily the symbol of the urge to become aware, to understand and integrate unconscious intuition or five senses. Mercury in Cancer in a birth chart suggests a person who perceives through the unconscious and evaluates his perceptions through feeling. Mercury is the planet closest to the Sun, and is the Sun's messenger. The Sun is the symbol of essence, and Mercury is the symbol of that function which enables us to know essence.

Venus and Mars are another way of expressing Sun and Moon. "Venus is the urge to relate, harmonise and adjust in the sphere of personal relationships." "Mars is the urge toward conquest, separating and asserting self over others to fulfill desire." Mars desires. Venus is the urge to be desired.

The Moon is the mother, Venus is the archetype of the lover: these are the two faces of woman. The Sun is the father, Mars is the conqueror: these are the two faces of man.

The urge symbolised by Venus is expressed in the way a person adorns himself, his personal taste, his response to beauty, his social values, his values in relationships and what he seeks in the ideal partnership.

The urge symbolised by Mars is expressed in the way a person goes about getting what he wants, the quality or mode of his desire, the manner in which he chases it, and the expression of his passions.

For men, Mars is a more accessible energy, and for women. Venus is more accessible.

Jupiter and Saturn are the guardians at the gate of the personal world. They symbolise the urge to transcend the limited confines of the ego. Jupiter, a god of the heavens in mythology, is connected with the "upper" regions of the intuitive mind, while Saturn a god of the Earth, is connected with the "lower" regions of the personal unconscious, the dark side of human nature. Jupiter is a masculine urge, and Saturn is feminine.

Jupiter is concerned with the religious urge in man, the urge to experience the divine and create this experience through symbols. The sign in which Jupiter is placed in an individual's birth chart suggests the way in which he seeks this experience of meaning in life.

Saturn urges us to identify more and more with our limitations and our subjective interpretations of life, so that we eventually isolate ourselves so much that we are in a hell of dissociation from the deepest underlying currents of life. Through our pain, we become aware of that which is greater than the ego. In this way, Saturn is the great teacher.

Neptune, Uranus and Pluto are in the realm of the collective unconscious. The urges which these planets symbolise are rarely available to the consciousness of the individual.

Uranus and Neptune form another male-female pair. Uranus is the masculine pole and Neptune the feminine.

Uranus is the Awakener, "the urge to break free from identification with material reality and to experience the world of the archetypal mind." One may experience Uranus in the urge to change one's understanding of oneself, one's work, one's beliefs or one's relationships.

Neptune is a water deity, and although he is a male figure in mythology, the energy he personifies is feminine. "Neptune is a symbol of the sea of collective feeling which moves us from below to immerse ourselves in the mass, offering up our hard-won and precarious individuality so that we may purify ourselves through dissolution." We can see this energy operating in a low level in any mob, motivated by a single emotional focus. In its highest form, the symbol of Neptune is the urge for purification, the experience of cleansing through immersion in the sea of the collective unconscious a truly religious experience.

Neptune and Uranus are usually unconscious in the majority of individuals and are experienced as powerful events which seem to be caused by the external hand of fate. However, such events are attracted inevitably by the Nepturian and Uranian forces within the psyche.

Pluto in mythology was Lord of the Underworld, ruling the dead and the riches of the earth. "The Symbol of Pluto is concerned with the archetypal experience of beginnings and endings, death and rebirth." But death is only an illusion, for the cycle of perpetual change and renewal is endless. we experience Pluto in the sphere of relationships - in emotional deaths and the feeling of loss, and rebirth in new relationships. Pluto is also connected with sexuality - in that the sexual act symbolises the death of separateness in union. The procreation of a child causes a Plutonian change in the psyche ; from being a child, one has now become a parent. One phase has died and another is born. Pluto also rules the death of the physical body.

> *"The planets are symbols of the powers of the unconscious. "They symbolise archetypal experiences or energies which exist in all of life and exist also within man, who is part of life. Once we have learned to understand the energies they symbolise, we can seek to understand their meanings when placed in particular signs of the zodiac, in an individual's birth chart."*
>
> \- Lenni Foster

An understanding of the elements helps us to understand aspects (or energy connections between planets).

Fire and Air are considered active or positive, and Water and Earth are passive and receptive or negative.

The element Fire refers to Energy, and it exemplify high spirits, confidence in themselves, enthusiasm, inspiration, strength and a direct honesty. They may also be willful and impatient.

The element Air is compatible with Fire, and it refers to the Mind. Air signs see reality in terms of ideas, theories, concepts, thought and opinions, and can lack deep emotion.

The element Water refers to Emotion, feeling responses and sensitivity. At their highest, water signs can be psychically intuitive, and at their lowest, subject to compulsive desires, fears and emotional in stability.

The element Earth is compatible with Water and refers to the Physical Senses, the body, and the reality of the material world. Earth signs rely on practical reason and are usually more patient, cautious and self-disciplined than the other signs, but can also lack imagination and be unable to deal with the abstract realms.

The element of the Sun sign (e.g. the Sun in Taurus is in the element Earth) reveals the attunement of one's basic vitality and the fundamental quality of one's consciousness. The fire signs are motivated by their inspirations and aspirations, the earth signs by their material needs, the air signs by intellectual concepts, and the water signs by their deepest emotional yearnings.

The element of our Sun sign is the source of our basic vitality, and the power which enables us to revitalize ourselves in order to cope with the stresses and demands of daily life.

The Moon relates to the unconscious, so the element of the Moon sign will indicate inner drives and desires, also instinctual reactions.

The Ascendant influences the way we deal with our environment, the way we project ourselves and the immediate impressions that others may have of us.

To Look at an example, a woman with her Sun in Scorpio (a water sign) Moon in Libra (air) and Capricorn Ascendant (earth) may seem on the surface, because of the Ascendant, to be at ease with the demands of practical reality, but the intensely emotional Sun (water element) will be more fundamental to her sense of reality and she will also experience the more unconscious, instinctual drive of the Moon to evaluate everything objectively, be detached and think before acting (air element). In this example, the woman would feel some conflict because air and water are not compatible elements - water wanting emotional expression and air wanting to stop and think first.

It means that if we are basically an air/water person, we should continue to express ourself through thoughts and emotions, but also be aware of the energy and direction of fire, and the practical material strength of earth, and try to be open to the validity of these elements.

There is a part of our mind which correlates with our thoughts and emotions to identify to such an extent that we even say "I am happy" or "I am in despair". If however we can detach ourselves and stand back from the drama of our own egos, we can see that it is really more accurate to say, "My emotions are happy" or "My mind has had a thought" for that part of us that watches is not the ego.

So far we have learnt that the 3 essential steps of the Alchemical process are:

1. Seperation
2. Purification
3. Cohobation

We are all familiar with what this means in the physical laboratory, but it will also prove useful to try and understand what these 3 processes mean in the Microcosm.

By the Microcosm, we mean Man itself, the inner Man, his soul or consciousness.

The Macrocosm being all that which lies outside of the body of Man.

It is essential to understand and Work the 3 steps in the Microcosm and Macrocosm simultaneously.

Since if one aspires to the perfection of the Philosopher's Stone, it cannot be made materially in the Macrocosm until the Microcosm turns into Philosopher's Stone.

Separation in the Microcosm means the removal of our identification of Self with our ego and the identification of Self with our source or God.

Thus the separation is from our ego or that part of us which identifies with the duality of the material world with its associated beliefs and emotions.

Paradoxically, this separation leads to a union. When operating from the Higher Self there is no identification with negative emotions or with prejudicial belief structures and the Self can then operate in the material world with clear sight (clairvoyance). When one is in this state of consciousness, it could be said that one is in this world but is not of this world.

Separation can take many forms and shapes and is practiced in all religions in a great variety of disciplines of the mind, body and emotions. These methods attempt to contact, utilize, evoke and develop the Higher Self within, at the same time quieting the emotions and beliefs of the Reactional Self or Ego.

A simple approach to self-observation is the exercise of the brain, whereby one attempts each day to separate or stand aside from oneself and see the World as an observer.

> *"If we become a little more free from the mutual exclusion of opposites and, instead of being at one pole or the other either being attracted or repelled, we will experience the force between them in ourselves. This is the force of life that lifts us out of the mechanical life and it is for this that the Reactional Self exists.*
>
> *Only when the opposites can be experienced together in us can we begin to be aware of our own human nature. This nature that we have is something with enormous depth and if we are caught by our reactions we are condemned to live only a surface existence; but if we can use the force of our reactions we have a way of penetrating to what lies within us. The rightful place of the Reactional Self is that of a generator of energies and the combination of opposites is that condition of transformation in which higher grades of energy can*

be produced Just as with electricity it is impossible to generate a current unless we have learnt how to separate the positive and negatives poles, so it is only when we have learnt how to separate the positive and negative forces of our Reactional Self that we can gain from our activities a source of energy for our inner work."

- John Bennett

"Alchemy is a process of evolution towards perfection, of a process of overcoming disease.

Disease in the mundane sense refers only to the physical body - the lack of integrity of its function thru infection, injury, etc. Looking further we see many suffering from mental illness today. Schizophrenia is a general name given to the majority of mental problems that one in ten Americans and Australians complain of and are treated for at least at one stage in their lives. Schizophrenia is defined by the Oxford Dictionary as "a form of mental disease in which the personality is disintegrated and detached from its environment; 'split mind' literally".

-The Man of the Zodiac: Wood engraving, Paris 1491

Hence, in disease we have a split, separation or disintegrity in our body and/or mind.

The separation is from our own core or God, for God is both our true inner core and the Natural world outside us.

Thus, those alienated from their environment are simultaneously alienated from themselves within.

"The Centre of the Cyclone is that rising quiet central low-pressure place in which one can learn to live eternally. Just outside this centre is the rotating storm of one's own ego, competing with other egos in a furious high-velocity circular dance. As one leaves centre, the roar of the rotating wind deafens one more and more as one joins this dance.

One's centred thinking-feeling-being, one's own Satoris, are in the centre only, not outside.

One's push-pulled driven states, one's anti-Satori modes of functioning, one's self-created hells, are outside the centre.

In the centre of the cyclone one is off the wheel of Karma, of life, rising to join the Creators of the Universe, the Creators of us. Here we find we have created Them who are us."

-John Lilly

Apart from seeing disease in terms of separation from the one or lack of wholeness, we may equally see disease as imbalance. In this case wholeness or perfection lies in balance. The created material and mental worlds exist by virtue of the Law of Polarity or Duality. Thus, we are surrounded by this principle of opposites. The Chinese Taoists spoke of Yin and Yang throughout the Created Universe. Disease will occur when an excess of one principle occurs or a deficiency of the other. An excess may take the form of tension, fear, over secretion of a gland, for example.

Only from the central point of balance may evolutionary growth take place. Only from the union of positive and negative may a new positive of a higher order arise.

All the above implies that Cure of Disease lies in focusing the life on God, or in integrating life with the focus on the evolution of consciousness; the expansion of potentials and the revelation of the higher self.

Paracelcian notion of disease is that disease is not caused by the stars as such, but there is a harmonic correspondence between certain planetary bodies and their respective human mental attributes and physical organs. The Macrocosmic (Astral) and the Microcosmic (Human) are reflections of the same principle; one is not subordinate to the other.

When any disturbance in life manifests or any pattern, any motion, any crisis, any important happening - it has both a physical and a psychic reflection, or both a microcosmic and macrocosmic reflection. One does not cause the other. Both occur synchronistically and are expressions of the one principle inherent in both. If we find ourselves under any astral influence, the stars are no more the cause of the influence than we or our Karmas are, but because we are bound by time, cause appears separated from effect.

The concept of the four humours of the Hermetic philosophy was related to the elements of astrology (fire-type = choleric; water-type = melancholic; air-type = phlegmatic; earth-type = sanguine).

This implied that excess of one element produced an individual of one of the above types. A healthy, well-balanced individual was said to need a balance of all the 4 elements.

This constitutional medicine is parallel to the Hindu theory of Tridosha.

> *"Diseases serve to teach man that he is made out of the universal Limbus (Nature), and that he is like the animals and by no means better than they. He should study himself and the rest of creation, so that he may obtain self-knowledge; and this self-knowledge should be above all obtained by the physician."*
>
> *"Why does man want to eat, to drink, and to breathe, but because he is related to the elements of the earth, water and air, and must attract these things to his constitution; why does he need warmth, but because he is related to the element of fire and cannot do without it, and all these elements may produce diseases.*
>
> *There is no disease in the elements, but the disease starts from the centres. The origin of diseases is in man, and not outside of man; but outside influences act upon the*

inside and cause disease to grow. A physician who knows nothing about Cosmology will know little about disease. He should know what exists in heaven and upon the earth, what lives in the four elements and how they act upon man; in short, he should know what man is, his origin and his constitution; he should know the whole man and not merely his external form.

If man were in possession of a perfect knowledge of self, he would not need to be sick at all."

- Johann Georg Gichtel

In the perspective of Tantra Philosophy, Man is the highest of all animals, he has the power to attain self-knowledge, a faculty which the animals do not possess. The three inherent qualities in Man; Satta, Tama and Raja or the three philosophical sensory nerves, Ida, Pingala and Sushumna or the constitutions Vata, Pitta and Kapha in the higher living organisms are the necessary ingredients for the Inner - Alchemical processes of the Soul or Prana or Life energy which is going on in the organisms. If for any internal or external causes this Inner-Alchemical process is interrupted, disease is occurred, and ceasation of this process paves the way for departure of the Soul from the physical body. Siddhars or Murshids (Al-Mu'in / Spiritual Master) or Alchemists who have achieved perfection in the art of controlling this Inner-Alchemy through repeated distillation of the Life energy (Vital fluid or effluence as per Franz Anton Mesmer) can attain Siddhi or have control over the Life span.

16

Fermentation & Distillation of Wine Spirit

One of the oldest chemical reactions utilized by man is fermentation- - the conversation of sugar in fruit juice into alcohol and carbon dioxide by the action of yeast. The fermentation of grape sugar is summerized by the below equation:

$C_6H_{12}0_6$ + Zymase → $2C_2H_5OH$ + $2CO_2$ + Zymase

in words

Glucose + Zymase from yeast → grain alcohol + carbon dioxide

The reaction will proceed until the alcohol content of the fermentation mixture rises to a certain level which destroys the yeast. At this point a solution is present which contains sugar, alcohol, and water is commonly called wine. (If the carbon dioxide is not allowed to escape, the solution is called champagne.) By separating the alcohol from the wine, other alcoholic beverages can be prepared which contain a higher alcohol content than wine.

In separating alcohol from wine, a chemist affects the separation of a liquid from a solution, and, this separation is executed by distillation. Distillation is based on the fact that the matter can exist in three phases ; solid, liquid and gas. As the temperature of a pure substance is increased, it passes through these phases, making a transition at a specific temperature from solid to liquid (melting point) and then at a higher temperature from liquid to gas (boiling point). Distillation involves evaporating a liquid into a gas phase, then condensing the gas back into a liquid and collecting the liquid in a clean receiver. Substances that have a higher boiling point than the desired material will not distill at the working temperature, and remain behind in the flask. Alcohol has a lower boiling point than water (and sugar) and thus distillation can separate the alcohol from the wine. Some water also evaporates, and the separation is not complete, hence wines are not pure alcohol and bottles of alcoholic beverages are labeled with the alcohol content or in percent by volume, while for distilled liquors the alcohol content is usually given in terms of a "proof" rating. Proof is equal to twice the percent by volume of alcohol.

Distilling the Spirit of Wine

In this procedure, wine will be distilled and the alcoholic content of the distillate determined.

Distillation

1. Obtain a thermometer distilling flask and condenser from the front of the room.
2. Assemble the distilling apparatus as shown in the figure (See figure).
3. Remove the thermometer and place a boiling chip and about 75ml of wine using a long-stem funnel into the distilling flask.
4. Turn on the cooling water and have the instructor check your setup, then apply the heat to the wine. After boiling begins, reduce the heat so the wine boils at a moderate rate.
5. Watch the temperature closely while distilling and collect the distillate coming from the condenser while the temperature is in the range 80-85^{0}C. The temperature should remain nearly constant in this range.

6. When the temperature rises above 85 ^{o}C, begins to increase, quickly change collecting flasks then continues distilling until the temperature is between 98 and 100 ^{o}C.
7. Record the temperature range over which you collected the alcohol enriched distillate.

   Determination of alcohol content of the distilled spirit.
8. Determine the density of the brandies collected by weighing a known volume of each.
9. From the table of density versus percent alcohol and the result of step 8, determine the alcohol content of the distilled spirit. Record your result.

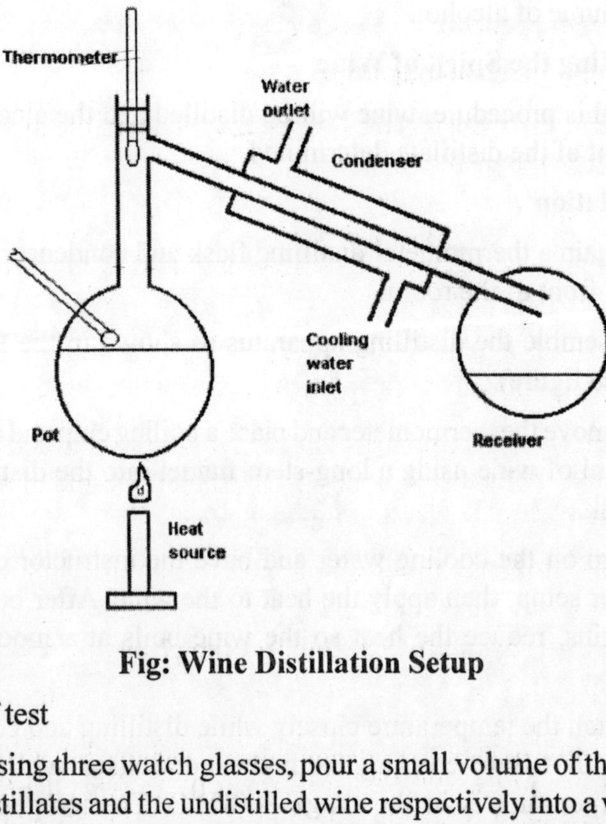

Fig: Wine Distillation Setup

Proof test

10. Using three watch glasses, pour a small volume of the two distillates and the undistilled wine respectively into a watch glass. Record the contents of each watch glass and then try

lighting the liquid with a wooden splint. Record whether the liquid in each watch glass burns or does not burn. Alcohol burns with a very faint blue flame. Extinguish with cold water.

Report Sheet for Distillation of Wine

Name____________Lab section__________ Date_______

Type of wine used____________

% Alcohol in wine (see label on bottle)____________%

Density of distilled spirit

a) Via hydrometer reading:__________%

b) Via measurement and calculation

Weight of graduated cylinder + distilled spirit: _________g

Weight of graduate cylinder: __________g

Weight of distilled spirit: __________g

Volume of distilled spirit in cylinder: __________ml

Density of distilled spirit __________g Ml

__________g /ml

Alcohol in distilled spirit in % (from table):____________

17

Spagyric Experiments

Experiment 1

Making Spagyric extract of Vitis Vinifera (Black Grape)

1. *Materials needed:*

   a. Vitis Vinifera leaves, fruits (4 ounces)

   b. Pure grain alcohol, 1 pint

   c. Distilled water, 1 quart

   d. Medium-sized pot with a tight-fitting lid or metal bowl

   e. Percolation cone or filter

   f. Collecting bowl

   g. Mason jar

   h. Heat source for boiling water

   i. An eyedropper

   j. Flameproof cast iron pot, open fire and vent (for calcinations)

2. *Refining the Mercury*

a. Mercury is universal in the plant world- that is, the distillate from fermented corn or other grains is chemically and alchemically identical to the pure distillate of fermented Vitis Vinifera.

b. What remains is to extract the chemical constituents of Vitis Vinifera using the grain alcohol (Mercury) in a percolation apparatus.

Note: Percolation is done only when the leaves are not fresh or dried.

c. First, thoroughly moisten 2 ounces of Vitis Vinifera leaf with 8 ounces of grain alcohol.

d. Next, pour 8 more ounces of alcohol into the percolation apparatus. Green extract should begin to drip into the collecting bowl. When you have 8 ounces of extract, the percolation is complete (may require some squeezing).

e. Set the extract aside in the mason jar. This is your Mercury of Vitis Vinifera.

3. Refining the Sulfur

a. Sulfur is the individual "personality" of the herb you are extracting: its smell, its flavor, its experience, and its soul. It obviously then varies from plant to plant, and is usually embodied in the essential oil.

b. We can isolate some of the essential oil using a simple steam distillation system.

c. Take the remaining 2 ounces of Vitis Vinifera fruits, pulverize it in a mortar and pestle, and place it in the bottom of the cooking pot. Place your now empty collecting bowl in the middle of the pot.

d. Pour just enough distilled water to cover the Vitis Vinifera into the pot, taking care not to get any in the collecting bowl.

e. Place the lid or metal bowl on the pot upside-down, and apply heat. Allow the pot to simmer only five minutes, then turn off the heat and wait for it to cool.

f. When the pot is cool, remove the lid and look in the collecting bowl. There should be a mixture of water and oil in it; draw it into the dropper and wait for the oil to rise to the top (this may take a little patience). Squeeze out the excess water, and add the oil to the mason jar. This is your Sulfur of Vitis Vinifera.

4. Refining the Salt through calcination

a. Salt is the tether, the connection to the physical plane, which is also unique to each herb you process. It represents the refined physical emanation of the plant, its "body", the vessel that Vital Force chose to incarnate into and, along with the Sulfur, animate.

b. The Salt is embodied in the soluble salts of the herb, which are extracted through calcination and subsequent evaporation.

c. The first step is to collect all the Vitis Vinifera you used so far and place it in the flameproof cast-iron pot.

d. Next, apply strong heat to the pot either outdoors, under a hood, or in a fireplace. There will be a good amount of smoke generated as the Peppermint burns.

e. It may be wise to cover the pot with a good lid, to prevent any ashes or too much smoke from escaping. After a few hours, the Vitis Vinifera should be burned down to a white ash. Stirring is helpful to ensure complete calcination.

f. Remove the ash, place it in the bottom of a separate vessel (ideally clear glass) and add 4 ounces of distilled water.

g. Allow the "death's head" (caput mortuum) to fall out of solution. These are the insoluble salts. When a clear liquid remains above the death's head, decant it into your collecting bowl.

h. Evaporate the liquid from your collection bowl either in a slow (150°) oven, or in the sunlight. You should be left with a white crystalline, salty residue. This are the soluble salts of the herbs you used for extraction, serving the biochemical purpose of hydrating cells and dispersing the extract into the far corners of the body, and the alchemical purpose of Salt of Vitis Vinifera.

i. Pulverize the Salt in a mortar and pestle, and add it to the mason jar.

5. The spagyric extract of Vitis Vinifera is complete! Label it and place it for storage in a cool, dark place or bottle as needed.

Experiment 2

Making of Spagyric Elixir

To create spagryic elixirs, the following equipment is required:

1 Mason Jar

1 Mortar and Pestle

1 Knife

1 Long glass rod or metal spoon

1 Plant, chosen according to Planetary correspondence

1 One bottle of approximately 700 ml Alcohol distilled from wine (Spirits of Wine).*

1 Litre of distilled water

1 Flask with stopper

1 500 ml pyrex flask with neck and spherical base (see image above on right)

2 500 ml pyrex vessels or beakers (measuring cups)

1 Retort w/tripod (see image above on left)

1 Butane burner w/fuel

1 Heating apparatus: a gas stove, alternatively a electric hot plate

1 Balneum Arenae - a sand bath**

1 Glass funnel

1set of Filtering Paper-lab grade, alternatively coffee filters

1 ceramic dish (resistant to very high temperatures) with lid (Crucible)

1 large cloth of linen

Note: *The Menstruum or Alkahest (i.e. the mercurial spirit) must consist of Spirits of Wine or Grappa.

**To prepare a sand bath, acquire a fine grained sand (for example as used in a aquarium) and pour it into in a large metallic heat resistant vessel.

1. Distil one litre of water using a simple retort on a tripod and butane burner. Store the distilled water in an air sealed flask and in darkness.
2. Choose a Plant- the First Matter (Materia Prima)- According to the desired effect according to Planet and/or accepted quality of the plant. Pluck the plant by its roots during its corresponding Planetary day and hour. (Frater Albertus in his Practical Laboratory Alchemy recommends to alternatively pick the plant during sunrise on the Day the Planet rules. Should you wish to work with a Plant's Elemental energies, simply pick the plant during the appropriate elemental tide. Astrological energies may be accessed by picking the plant when the Sun is in the house of the Sign you wish to work with. He further states that this plant is Isis, in it's Virginal State, i.e. before plucking).

   Select a time which is favourable according to the dignities of the planets, aspects, etc.

   Gather the plucked plant into a airtight jar and put it concealed from the sun.

The following table should help explain some of the planetary influences climatic changes especially in the weather during summer and winter. A careful observation over a greater length of time and a conciencious record kept would prove valuable for further calculations concerning lunar influences.

Change of Moon* Between the hours of:	Summer	Winter
Midnight - 2:00 A.M.	Fair	Strong frost; partly windy
2:00- 4:00 A.M.	Cool; sometimes storm indications	Snow and wind
4·:00- 6:00 A.M	Rain; uncertain	Rain or snow
6:00- 8:00 A.M	Windy; part rain	Strong winds
8:00- 10:00 A.M	Very Changeable	Cold rain and snow
10:00- 12:00 A.M	Changeable, inclined to stormy weather	Cold wind
Noon - 2: 00 P.M	Rain	Snow and Rain
2:00 P.M. 4:00 P.M	Very Changeable	Unsteady; getting warmer
4:00- 6:00 P.M	Fair	Dry and cold
6:00- 8:00 P.M	Windy	Cold wind; some snow
8:00 10:00 P.M	Windy	Windy, cold; little snow
10:00 - Midnight	Fair	Fair and cold

*This represents the various phases of the moon such as Full, New, First, or Last Quarter Moon. Where the particular moon phases take place is not alone sufficient to determine the changes, since they occur in various signs of the Zodiac. Therefore a New Moon taken alone in a sign is not the exact indication of an indicated change, rather it is the time when the particular moon phase commences. This means at what time it takes place and in what sign which will tell the observer what shall occur. Planetary influences is discussed in details in the companion book Pharmacodynamics in Alkemi-Spagyric Medicine.

3. Spread out the plant over a folded out newspaper. Let it dry in a moderate temperature and away from the rays of the sun. Let it dry for at least a week. Then put it into the air tight jar again as before.

4. Prepare your Oratory (your Temple space) as in the 0°=0° Grade on the Day of the Planet corresponding to the plant. Place the jar filled with the herb, together with the empty Mason Jar, mortar and pestle, and bottle with the Spirits of Wine on the Altar. Enter into the Oratory and work if possible by candle light from this point onward. Put on your robes and insignia. Perform banishings, purifications and consecrations of Hall and invocation of the Highest Divine Force. Do a preliminary invocation (i.e. the Opening by Watchtower) if an Adept. On the Planetary Hour, invoke the Planetary Force using the appropriate rites and implements. State the intention, i.e. the Goal of the Work. Perform a Middle Pillar Ritual.

5. Use a knife blessed ritually for this purpose, and chop the plant into parts as small as you can make them. Whilst doing this, have a prayerful state of mind, and envision the Goal of the work. Also be mindful of your Middle Pillar and draw Light down the Pillar to Malkuth when you inhale and up to Tiphareth and out through your hands while you exhale. Frater Albertus also recommends using your breath to inhale the Light, and as you exhale, sending a cloud of the Light via visualisation and the will to surround the First Matter that you are working with (the plant). He further states that the work of Alchemy takes place on multiple levels at once - In the Soul (Sulphur), Spirit (Mercury), and the Salt (Body). It is important that you conduct the

work with full awareness of this. Following recipes for herbal tinctures/plant Stones without utilizing the energy of Light or the concentrative powers of the mind is fruitless.)

6. Having chopped the First Matter as finely as possible you now place the matter into the Mortar and grind it in parts with the Pestle. Again remember to focus strongly on the goal, and project the Light into the First Matter as you exhale.

Maceration

7. When it is ground as fine as you can make it, take the matter and place it in the Mason Jar. Pour the Spirits of Wine over the matter, until the alcohol is twice as high in the jar as the top of the matter. It is important to leave some air in the Jar, as the process of Maceration requires Air to enable a continuous circulation within the flask (i.e. the vaporization and the following liquidization) - a process of sublimation of the essence (i.e. Sulphur and Mercury) and subsequent cohobation. In this process the Soul and Spirit of the plant (its Sulphur and Mercury) are separated from the body (its Salt) through the agency of the Solvent or transferative medium (the Spirits of Wine - which also is a Mercury), i.e. the Alkahest or Menstruum.

8. Do another invocation over the Mason Jar. Trace a circle round it and then the appropriate Hexagrams, Hebrew characters and sigils. Purify with Water and Consecrate with Fire as in the opening. Cover and wrap the Jar with a sheet of linen (Frater Albertus recommends covering the mason jar with Aluminium foil, which he sees as severely diminishing the penetration of mental currents. He believes this is a good thing, as the matter and its Essence will be very sensitive and receptive to mental and astral currents during it's fermentation. Personally believe this to be somewhat overkill. The linen will do fine.)

9. Set the wrapped Mason Jar in a moderately warm place (i.e. of normal room temperature), where it will not be disturbed. (Frater Albertus adviced to set it high up, where the Light of the Sun will warm it, without people disturbing it. The warmth enables the expansion and contraction, which in turn allow the separation and concentration to take place. Personally I believe there is no need to expose the Mason Jar and its contents in temperatures beyond 20° C.) Leave the Tincture within the dark womb of the Mason Jar for as many weeks as the corresponding Planetary number (if you for example have chosen a Plant sacred to Jupiter, it should be in maceration for four weeks, if sacred to Venus, for seven weeks, etc.)
10. On each Planetary Day (with a weekly interval), and on its Planetary Hour, take out the Mason Jar and unwrap it. Shake it gently with large circulating (clockwise) movements. Put it again on the Altar and perform an additional Planetary invocation. Repeat the invocation over the Mason Jar, purify and consecrate, etc. Rewrap it and put it away again.

Separation

11. At the appropriate Planetary Day and Hour, take out the Mason Jar and unwrap it. Put it on the Altar and perform an additional Planetary invocation. Repeat the invocation over the Mason Jar, purify and consecrate, etc. Now open the Jar. The liquid will be Dark, as it has absorbed the Life of the plant.
12. Separate the Sulphur and Mercury away from the Salt. This is done by putting the funnel into a flask. Put a filtering paper in the funnel and pour the macerated solution over it; the essence (Sulphur & Mercury) will pour into the flask while the Salt will remain in the filter. Squeeze out all liquid from the filter. Put a stopper on the flask containing this part of the Elixir - the tincture. (Frater Albertus

recommends vibrating HARP-PAR-KRATES* and using the Sign of Silence at this juncture, envisioning the flask surrounded in a blue mist, preventing the penetration of the flask (and thus the tincture) by unwanted thought forms. It seems like a good idea and a nice addition). Put away the flask into a cabinet sealed from light; let no sunlight enter into the tincture at this juncture.

*Shaman's magical para-phernalia musical bow, rasp, rattle or harp.

Calcination

13. Take up the dead matter - caput mortum - of the plant, and having placed it within your ceramic container (Crucible), place it upon your heating apparatus. Incinerate the matter with a match, so that the Salt may be refined into it's purest and living state by burning off the dead matter. (Frater Albertus comments: "Remember here the INRI* of the Analysis of the Key Word ritual. Igne Natura Renovatur Integra in Fire, Nature is perfectly renewed!") The alcohol of your Mercury should fuel this burn for some time. Take the glass rod or spoon and poke the dead matter with it so that it will burn thoroughly. When it has finished burning - i.e.. when all the alcohol has been combusted - turn on the stove at full heat and let the matter burn into a black ash. This process is called Cineration. (Note: The process of Cineration will emit lots of smoke, so take care to provide with good ventilation while you perform it.) When it is finished turn off the heat and let everything cool down.

*INRI stems from the Latin phrase 'Iesus Nazarenus Rex Iudaeorum' meaning 'Jesus of Nazareth, King of the Jews'.

14. Place the ash it in the Mortar and grind it down to a fine powder with the Pestle. Then pour it again in the ceramic container, put on the lid and place it on the stove anew and at full heat. Let it now burn into a grey ash. This may take several hours before you turn of the heat. Remember to

use the most intense heat that you can apply. This is the process of Calcination proper.

15. Place the grey ash in the Mortar and grind it down again to a fine powder with the Pestle. Then pour it in the ceramic container and place it again on the stove and at full heat. Let it calcinate into a white ash, for as many hours as is necessary. When you are satisfied with the colour, turn of the heat and grind the white ashes with Mortar and Pestle. Scrape this off into a container and save it. The goal is to create as much white ash - the perfectly refined Salt (i.e. purified from the caput mortum) - as possible. (Frater Albertus comments: "The entire process above is Apophis, the separation, the Destroyer. When this is completed, once more say a prayer and enter a meditative state. Contemplate the refined and Seperated parts of the Plant. They are Osiris Slain.") But the refinement of the Salt doesn't end here. The purification of Salt must use both fire and water. After calcination (consecration with fire) of the Salts you must purify them with Water. This is done through filtering and "leaching".

Leaching

16. To do this critical process you must use your distilled water. Fill a measuring cup (the pyrex vessel called a beaker) with distilled water and mix the calcinated Salts in the water (stirring with a glass rod or spoon). Then take a funnel and put another filter on it. Then pour the water through it and into another pyrex measuring cup or beaker. Make sure to press all water from the filter. Repeat this process (with new filters each time) until there is no longer any residue in the filter. The resultant must now be in one of the two pyrex vessels and the Salt fully dissolved in the distilled water (stir with the glass rod or spoon to make sure).

17. Then leach the filtered water. This is done by putting the glass vessel on a moderated heat (on the radiator for example, or putting the vessel in the sandbath and everything on the stove, using the lovest possible heat) and let the water evaporate until nothing remains but white Salt crystals. If they are not remaining white (i.e. discoloured) you may calcinate again and purify with water and leach anew. This is important. The Salt must be crystallic and pure white. Now you are ready for the coagula phase, i.e. of mixing the Salts with the essence (Mercury and Sulphur).

Digestion

18. Repeat the invocation as before (on the Planetary Day and Hour) and now recombine the separated and refined parts (the three Alchemical Principles of Sulphur, Mercury and Salt) into the pyrex flask (spherical with neck - the philosophical egg); put the Salt crystals in the flask and pour over it the combined essence (Sulphur & Mercury, or to use Frater Albertus's words: "The Mercury carries the Sulphur within it's Womb"). Seal it hermetically with a stopper and stir the mixture, not with the rod or spoon but with gentle circulating (deosil) movements.

19. Again repeat the invocation over the flask, purify and consecrate, etc. Now place the flask in the prepared sand bath, and put everything on the stove and on the lowest possible temperature; the ideal temperature for digestion is approximately the temperature of the human body, not over 40° and not below 35° Celsius. Let it now digest for as many weeks as the Planetary number. If you aspire to produce a Plant Stone, instead of a Elixir, you could instead multiply the number of weeks by the number of the Planet. (Frater Albertus recommends letting it rest for at the very least one week, and preferably for one entire Moon Cycle, "so that the mixture may gestate, and the Mercury further

absorb the qualities of both the Sulphur and of the refined Salt". He further recommends an altogether different method compared to mine (and I cite him): "After this time [of gestation] has passed, set up your retort, receiving flask (this can be any container, really. It needed be a lab flask [use the pyrex flask - S.R.]) and Butane burner. Enter once more into a meditative, and say a prayer of thanksgiving to the Deity. Pour the tincture into the retort, seal the top, and set the burner Alight. Now, the Mercury will rise from the tincture with the application of heat, and transfer to the receiving flask. Perform the Analysis of the Keyword ritual; during the final Vibration of Light, visualize a pillar of white light descending into the receiving flask and joining the Mercury. This Mercury will contain the refined Essence of the Plant - we have separated, refined, and re-combined the parts of the plant, so that the finished product is of much higher vibration. This new Mercury is the true Tincture, and contains Osiris Risen-treat it as such!" In this instance it is important to recombine the essence (i.e. Sulphur and Mercury) with the Salt again, i.e. perform a cohobation. This process is then repeated several times, as many times as the Planetary number. This is therefore a continuous sublimation and cohobation. Personally I believe that the distillation with retort isn't necessary at all, even though it creates wonderful symbology. It can suffice with the pyrex flask (hermetically sealed) and a moderate source of heat (around the normal temperature of the body) in several weeks, which will create a continuous "circulation" (i.e. a continuous sublimation and cohobation - but within the flask) which probably will make the elixir more potent and the following digestion perhaps even create the much sought after "plant stone".

20. After the set time has elapsed, ending on the Planetary Day and Hour, turn of the stove and remove the pyrex

flask from the sand bath. Remove the stopper and pour out the finished elixir or - by the grace of God - the Plant Stone. Place it within a specially marked bottle with stopper.

21. Take up a glass filled with mineral water and pour some drops into it using a pipet (Frater Albertus instead recommends distilled water and around 2 ml of the completed Tincture). Drink this Elixir, and then sit in meditation. Make careful record of the effects you feel in the physical and subtle bodies. You may experience visions as well, so take note of these. They will reveal much to you of the power invoked by the Elixir, and of the plant used in the Elixir it self. Afterwards take out the flask from the Oratory and store it in a dry and light sealed compartment.
22. Perform a banishing of the Planet in question, lesser banishings and a licence to depart.

Note: Take a few drops of the Elixir in mineral water each morning prior to breakfast. If you have managed to produce a Plant Stone, you will have to make the test: put it in the Crucible on the stove and on full heat. The solid stone will now melt into a wax. Turn off the heat and the wax will solidify into a Stone again. To use it, scrape of a tiny bit (a few grams) and dissolve it into the mineral water before drinking.

Experiment 3

Extraction of the Salt of Plants

Pick at least 5kg of Ocimum San or of another plant that you choose and dry it in the sun. After it becomes very dry, incinerate it on a sheet of iron.

Gather the ashes from the incineration, place them in an iron frying pan, and set the pan on a gas stove.

Adjust the stove to a very high heat and calcine the ashes for one hour, constantly stirring them with a stainless steel spoon. When the ashes are well calcined they will be a clear grey colour.

Next, pour 750 ml of rainwater into a 1 litre large-mouth flask. While they are still hot, add the ashes to the rainwater, a little at a time.

It is important that the water level is at least one hand's-width above the ashes. Add more water if necessary to reach the desired level. If one flask is not enough to hold all the water, divide the ashes between two or three flasks as necessary. Stir the water/ash mixture well with a glass rod and then let it settle for one hour.

If the ashes have been properly calcined, as our Art demands, the water of the lixiviation will be clear and transparent; otherwise, it will be the colour of tea.

In another similar flask, place a glass or plastic funnel with a small cotton lid. Decant the water of lixiviation* by pouring it into the funnel, and when everything has drained, add the ashes to the funnel with a stainless steel spoon. Rinse the original lixiviation flask with a little rainwater and pour it onto the ashes in the funnel. When the whole liquid has been drained, pour some more rainwater on the ashes to extract all of the soluble salt that remains in them.

*to extract a soluble constituent from (a solid mixture) by washing or percolation.

Pour the lixiviated liquid into a porcelain container and set it in a sand bath, which has been placed in an electric, or gas oven. As the water evaporates, the dissolved salt will begin to crystallize or coagulate, and as the evaporation proceeds further, a film will be created on the surface of the thickening liquid, which will impede the continued evaporation of the water.

Therefore, when the solution arrives at the point where it develops a surface film, we recommend stirring it well with a glass rod, to break-up the superficial layer of coagulated salt.

After all of the water has evaporated, the remaining coagulated salt should be as white as snow. If it is not white, you will have to calcine it again in a stainless steel porringer or pan, with a very strong fire and dissolve it in fresh rainwater once again, following the instructions given above. The secret to extracting the white salt the first time is the proper and complete calcination of the ashes. Do not be in a hurry in executing this operation, because if it is done properly, it will save you a great deal of work.

Conclusions

Write an essay to defend your choice of hypothesis. You will combine the information about the known properties of materials and vehicles used, with your experimental observations to support your hypothesis.

You may suggest further experiments that you could or would like to do to prove your hypothesis. Do not conduct any experiments without the prior approval of your teacher.

18

Explanation of Some Spagyrics Terms

Incineration

The conversion of a substance to ashes by means of a powerful fire.

The incineration of the plant material is to drive off the carbons and all superfluities to obtain the black ashes wherein is hidden our precious salts. Our sulfur is also driven off with this incineration however it will be reintroduced through the cohobation just prior to the distillation.

Calcination

The breaking down of a substance by fierce heating and burning usually in an open crucible.

Heat turns all black materials white. This is our calcination to remove the darkness from our matter. We can see the great amount of heat that develops in the impure black ash. The continuation of this heat is prolonged through several days as the dark colored ash turns into a light gray colored ash.

As our ashes become more and more light in color, so does the volume diminish as the impurities are continuously driven off back to their source in nature. When we are satisfied with the light colored of our ashes we then dissolve them in distilled water to separate the soluble salts from the insoluble salts.

Extraction of various fixed and unfixed sulphur fractions

Menstruum remains after extraction of Mercury is Sulphur, when it is properly dried and burned and calcined is called fixed.

Salts of Sulphur

Properly burned dried menstrum will be of whitish grey color, there may be color variations due to improper burn or impurities, in such cases the Salt yielded will not be of pure white color, and we have to repeat the process of burning the menstrum.

Calcination

The breaking down of a substance by fierce heating and burning usually in an open crucible.

Circulation

The purification of a substance by a circular distillation in a pelican or closed distillation apparatus. Through heating the liquid component separates, is condensed and descends again to the substance in the flask.

Cohobation

The frequent removal of the moist component of a substance by heating. Often the moist component (or some other liquid) is added and the process continued.

Crystallization

The formation of crystals out of a solution of the substance usually in water, either by their gradual formation from the liquid, or by evaporation of the liquid.

Digestion

The slow modification of a substance by means of a gentle heat.

Disintegration

The breaking down or dissociation of a substance into different parts.

Distillation

The separation of a volatile component from a substance by heating so as to drive off the component as a vapour which is condensed and collected in a cooler part of the apparatus.

Fermentation

The rotting of a substance, usually of an organic nature, often accompanied by the release of gas bubbles.

Fixation

To make a volatile subject fixed or solid, so that it remains permanently unaffected by fire.

Bibliography

1. Clerc, A., Die vereinfachte Medizin oder die ComplexeHomöopathie.H. Georg, Verlagsbuchhandlung Basel, 1892.
2. Droste, R., Komplexhomöopathie von Pastor Felke bis heute. Naturheilpraxis 3/2007.
3. Kenyon, J.,Die Medizin des 21. Jahrhunderts. Johannes Sonntag Verlagsbuchhandlung GmbH München 1990.
4. Liebau, K.F., Zur Komplexhomöopathie. Naturheilpraxis 02/2003.
5. Lutze, A., Lehrbuch der Homöopathie. Köthen: Lutze. 1860; Nachdruck: Heino Schirm (Hg.) 1978 München: Hieronymus (zitiert in Sahler).
6. Pascoe-Kompendium. Therapeutisches Handbuch und Präparateverzeichnis. 2007, Pascoe pharmazeutische Präparate GmbH.
7. Pharmacodynamics in Electro Homeopathy by Dr. Debasish Kundu (B Jain Publishers).
8. Materia Medica and Practice of Medicine in Electro Homeopathy by Dr. Debasish Kundu (Originals).
9. Pharmacodynamics in Spagyric Medicine (Plant Alchemy), Dr. Debasish & Sudeshna Kundu, Edited by Gisela Bruckel, (Germany), El Akrem Hayouni (Tunisia), Forworded by Dr. Peter Morrell (UK), (Originals).

10. Natural Medicines by Dr. Debasish Kundu & Dr. Malik A.K.Awan, Foreworded by Rui Olliviera (Kruger Brentt, U.K.).

11. Orders of The Great Work- Alchemy by Manly P. Hall, (P.R.S., Los Angeles, 1940).

12. The Golden Game: Alchemical Engravings of the Seventeenth Century, Stanislas Klassowski de Rolla, (Braziller, New York, 1988).

13. Jesse London Estrin, The Philosopher's Stone: A Study of the Quest for Perfection and Transmutationin the works of Paracelsus Theophrastus, Jesse London Estrin, Independently Published, April 2006.

14. Tantrasara Nirnaya, Gupta A, Shastri M. R, Sagar Press, Bombay, 1918.

15. Tantratattwa, Shibchandra Bidyarnab Bhattacharya, Nabbharat Publishers, Kolkata, 1972.

16. Kundalini: The Arousal of the Inner Energy, Ajit Mookerjee, Destiny Publishers, USA,1981.

17. Spagyric Medicine: Purification of Body, Mind and Spirit, Debasish Kundu, Alternative & Integrative Medicine Journal, http://www.omicsonline.org/scholarly-articles/spagyric-medicine-purification-of-body-mind-and-spirit-20111.html

18. Alchemy from Mystery to Medicine, Debasish Kundu, Homœopathic Links 2014; 27(2): 100-104.

19. Spagyric Homeopathy or Electro Homeopathy, Debasish Kundu, International Journal of Homeopathy & Natural Medicines, Vol. 1, No. 1, 2015, pp. 1-6. doi: 10.11648/j.ijhnm.20150101.11.

20. Count Cesare Mattei's Liquid Color Therapy, Sudeshna Kundu, Debasish Kundu, International Journal of Homeopathy & Natural Medicines. Vol. 1, No. 3, 2015, pp. 28-34. doi: 10.11648/j.ijhnm.20150103.11.

21. Sahler, A. M., Homöopathische Komplexmittel. Ihre historische Entwicklung, ihre Begründer und ihre gegenwärtige Bedeutung. Richard Pflaum Verlag, 2003.

22. Schauer, U., Zusammenfassung der klinischen Studie Antimigren, Pascoe pharmazeutische Präparate GmbH.

23. Schimmel, H. W., Die klinische Komplexhomöopathie. Der Versuch einer Definition. Acta biologica XXX/1, S.19, 1991.

24. Schimmel, H., Ursprung und geschichtlicher Abriss der Komplexhomöopathie. Acta biologica I/1 S. 5, 1962.

25. Stutz, E., Komplexhomöopathie: gestern, heute, morgen. Naturheilpraxis 3/2006.

26. Stutz, E., Tief sind die Wurzeln der Komplexhomöopathie. Naturheilpraxis 4/2004.

27. Albertus, Frater, The Alchemist's Handbook, Weiser Books (1974).

28. Greer, John Michael, Inside a Magical Lodge, Llewellyn (1998).

29. Junius, Manfred M., The Practical Handbook of Plant Alchemy, Healing Arts Press (1979).

30. Philalethes, Eirenaeus, Collectanea Chemica: Being Certain Select Treatises on Alchemy and Hermetic Literature, Alchemical Press (September 1991).

31. Stavish, Mark, The Path of Alchemy, Llewellyn Publications (2006).

32. Miller & Miller, A Guide to Personal Transformation, Miller & Miller, Phanes Press (1994).

33. Manfred M. Junius, Spagyrics: The Alchemical Preparation of Medicinal Essences, Tinctures, and Elixirs (Healing Arts Press, ISBN 1-59477-179-0).

34. Brian Cotnoir, Alchemy, Weiser, ISBN 1-57863-379-6.

35. The Medicinal Plant Industry, R. O. B. Wijesekera, CRC, (1991).

36. Stephen Arroyo, Astrology, Psychology and the Four Elements, CRCS Publication, USA, 1975.

37. An Astrological Guide to Living with Others on a Small Planet, by Liz Greene. A.H. & A.W. Reed Ltd. New Zealand & Australia, Samuel Weiser New York, 1978.

38. The Life and Doctrines of Paracelsus By Franz Hartmann. M.D., 1891/1963.

39. Theosophia Practica By Johann Georg Gichtel, ReInk Books (2014).

40. Jansky, R.C. How to Use the Cell Salts. Astro-Analytics Publications: Van Nuys, California, 1977.

41. P.D. Ouspensky, Tertium Organum: A Key to the Enigmas of the World, Aziloth Books, 2016.

Internet Resources Used:

Alchemy: https://en.wikipedia.org/wiki/Alchemy

Spagyrics: https://en.wikipedia.org/wiki/Spagyric

The Complete Great Work Photographed
http://www.rexresearch.com/caro/caro.htm

Star Fire: The Gold of the Gods
http://www.nexusmagazine.com/articles/starfire1.html

Lost Secrets of the Sacred Ark
http://www.nexusmagazine.com/articles/lostark.html

The History of Alchemy in America
http://www.hermetic.com/stavish/alchemy/history.html

High Alchemy - http://www.asc-alchemy.com/gold.html

Utopia in America - Sub Rosa Issue 3
http://subrosa.dailygrail.com

National Secrets - Atlantis Rising Issue 50
http://www.atlantisrising.com

The Chymistry of Isaac Newton, http://www.chymistry.org

Rasa Vidya, http://www.shrifreedom.com/alchemy.html

The Flow of Soma, http://www.vedanet.com

The Milky Way and the Cosmic Soma,
http://www.vedanet.com

The Ka, the Ba, and the Kabbalah
http://www.jayweidner.com/KaBa.htm

Secrets of Divine Lovemaking
http://www.geocities.com/alchematron/secretsofdivinelove.pdf

Seven Alchemy Formulas of Immortality
http://www.healingtaousa.com,
tao_alchemy_formulas.html

Notes on Spagyrics

By Dr. Debasish Kundu

Rs. 395/- US $ 21.50 Paperback

In this book author briefly discusses the principles of Alchemy with some exceptional notes on Sexual and Spiritual Alchemy.

CONTENTS: Note to the Readers, Foreword, Preface, Introduction, History of Alchemy, Spagyrics, Principles of Spagyrics, The Quest for the Quintessence, Plant Alchemy, Energetic Spagyrics, The Three Philosophical Principles, Spagyric Electro-Homoeopathy, Energy in the Organism, Herbal Medicine, Spiritual Alchemy, Sexual Alchemy, Spagyric Meditation, Hermetic Philosophy, Fermentation and Distillation of Wine Spirit, Spagyric Experiments, Explanation of Some Spagyrics Terms, Bibliography

Materia Medica and Practice of Medicine in Electro-Homoeopathy

By Dr.Debasish Kundu

Rs. 395/- US $ 21.50 Paperback

CONTENTS: Foreword, Preface, Electrohomoeopathy-An Introduction, Life History of Count Cesare Mattei, Preparation of Electro Homoeopathic Remedies, Electrohomoeopathy Formulas, Constitution and Temperament, Materia Medica of Electrohomoeopathy Medicines, Examination of the Patient, General Rules for Using the Medicines, Practice of Medicine, Points for External Application, Chief Points and their Uses, Clinical Index, Bibliography

Treatise on Spagyric Homoeopathic Pharmacy

By Dr. Debasish Kundu & Dr. Vijay Kant Agnihotri, Sr. Scientist, CSIR, Foreworded By Prof. Raffaele Pezzani, University of Padova, Italy

Rs. 395/- US $ 21.50 Paperback

It features all necessary information about the method of preparations and formulations of Zimpel, Krauss and Bernus. It is the only book which has incorporated Spagyrics formulas of Zimpel brought back from the lost fragments of time.

According to Prof. Pezzani, it is definitely a valuable guide, a friend that every Electrohomeopathy (according to Mattei) practitioner should possess. It is a must have collection for everyone.

CONTENTS: Dedication, Foreword, Preface, Spagyric Homeopathic Pharmacy, Electrohomoeopathy Formulas, Spagyrics after Zimpel, Krauss and Bernus, Medicinal Plants, Tables of Essential Oil Yielding Plants, Bibliography

Materia Medica for the New Age Man

By Dr. Debasish Kundu, Dr A.Jayasuriya, Chancellor, The Open International University, Colombo and Edited by Dr. M Ahmed, Member, Bangladesh Homeopathy Board, Dhaka

Rs. 450/- US $ 24.50 Hardbound

This is the only book which covered all therapeutic schools of Homeopathy, from Gemmotherapy, Lithotherapy, Bach flower to Spagyric Homeopathy.

CONTENTS: Foreword to the Second Edition, Introduction, Introduction to Homeopathy, Evolution of Disease, Introduction to Vital Force, Miasms, Homeopathic Pharmacy, Case Taking, Doctrine of Dosage, Therapeutic Schools of Homeotherapeutics at a Glance, Nosodes and Sarcodes, Materi^ Medica, Clinical Index of Homeopathic Remedies, Mother Tinctures (External Use), Do's and Don'ts for Patients, Clinical Tips for Dummies, General Index of Remedies, References

Treatise on Electro-Homoeopathic Pharmacy

By Dr. Debasish Kundu & Dr.Ajit Singh, Forewordeded By Prof. Fabio R Ambrosi, Chairman, Mattei Archieves, Italy

Rs. 195/- US $ 15.50 Paperback

CONTENTS: Foreword, Preface, Introduction to Electro Homoeopathic Pharmacy, Laboratory Equipments Used in Electro Homoeopathy Pharmacy, Vehicles used in Electrohomoeopathy, Sources of Electro Homoeopthic Medicines, Collection of Medicinal Plants, Cohobation: An Extraordinary Pharmacy, Methods of Preparation of Spagyric Medicines, Quality Control Procedures, Pharmacodynamics of Electrohomoeopathy Essences, Dosages and Mode of Administration, List of Medicinal Plants Used in

Electrohomoeopathic Remedies, Appendix 1: Terminology, Appendix 2: Prescription Writing, Appendix 3: Biographies, Appendix 4: Apparatus, Bibliography

Essentials of Acupuncture

By Dr. Debasish Kundu & Prof. Choo Led Sin, Chairman, International Federation of Acupuncture, Singapore

Rs. 995/- US $ 40.00 Hardbound

The Only Book which deals with Acupuncture Anaesthesia

CONTENTS: Preface, Introduction, History of Acupuncture, Philosophy of Acupuncture, Five Elements Theory, Diagnosis in Traditional Chinese Medicine, Evaluation and Diagnosis, The Concept of Qi, Management & Research on Some Disorders, How Acupuncture Works, Acupuncture Anesthesia, Laser Acupuncture, Auriculotherapy, Atlas of Acupuncture Points, Therapeutics of Common Ailments, Therapeutics of Common Ailments, Infertility, Impotence and Acupuncture, Acupuncture in Hairfall, Does Acupuncture Hurts, Related Therapies, Explanation of Some Terms, Marmapuncture, Bibliography

Cesare Mattei's Principles of Electro Homeopathy

Interpreted & Revised By Dr. Debasish Kundu

Rs. 395/- US $ 21.50 Paperback

The classic text has been Rewritten in simple language with much needed Interpretation & Revision. In some places the original French edition has been consulted, also enriched with footnotes wherever necessary.

CONTENTS: Preface by Editor, What is Electro-Homeopathy?, Names of the Electro-Homeopathic Remedies, General Information about the Electro-Homeopathic Remedies, Sphere of Action of the Remedies in Globules, General Remarks on the Electric Liquids, Their Mode of Application, Results of Experience, Doses and Method of Administration of the Remedies in Globules, Of Diagnosis, Principles and Rules for the Selection of the Appropriate Remedy, Easy Experiments for Beginners, Catalogue of Diseases Cured by Electro-Homeopathy, Appendix

Stepping Stones to Electo-Homoeopathy (Count Mattei's System of Medicine)

By A J L Gliddon(Original Edition with Vitiation of Blood and Lymph Theory)

Rs. 395/- US $ 21.50 Paperback

A brief insight into the discovery of electro homeopathy together with a rational explanation of the principles involved and the proposed medicines.

CONTENTS: Introduction , The Human Body, Count Mattei's Theories, Symptoms of Disease, The Electro-Homceopathic Remedies, The Globule Remedies, The Electricities, External Use of Electricities, External Use of Globules, Baths, Compresses, etc., How to Select the Remedies, How to Determine the Dose, Dilutions, Dry Globules, Table of Doses, Minute Doses, Effects of the Remedies, Other Hygienic Helps, Diet, Dress, Pure Air, etc.

Essentials of Trace Elements & Biochemic Medicine

By Prof. Dr. Debasish Kundu, Edited By Prof. Seyed Farzin Hassanzadeh Salehian Ph.D. (Iran)

Rs. 350/- US $ 19.00 Paperback

Cell Salts or Bioplasgens have always been considered an important part of healing in Homeopathy and Spagyrics. This book contains all essential materials concerning Trace Elements & Bioplasgen and their relationship with Spagyrics, Clinical Materia Medica with useful suggestions.

CONTENTS: Preface, Introduction to Trace Elements & Bioplasgens, The Functions of The Cell, Astrology and Bioplasgens, Minerals, Trace Elements, Materia Medica of the Bioplasgens, Bio-combinations, Bibliography

A Textbook on Food, Nutrition and Dietetics

By Dr. Debasish Kundu Editor Dr. Malik A.K. Awan Ph.D. (London), Associate Editor Prof. Seyed Farzin Hassanzadeh Salehian Ph.D.(Iran)

Rs. 495/- US $ 20.00 Paperback

CONTENTS: Preface, Relationship between Food, Nutrition & Health, History of Nutrition, Functions of Food, Digestion of Food, Food and Nutrition, Nutrition, Diet & Development, Nutrition & Diet Therapy, Nutrition for Infants, Children, Adults, Women and Elderly, Ideal Diet Plan, The Food Pyramid, Therapeutic Diet, Bibliography

Notes on MJT (Forensic Medicine & Toxicology)

By Dr. Debasish Kundu Ph.D. Assisted By Dr. Ravi Justin Raj NMD, LLB Edited By Dr. Malik A.K. Awan B.S., M.S. (Psychology), D.C.L., D.D. (U.S.A.), Ph.D. (London)

Rs. 550/- US $ 22.00 Paperback

CONTENTS: Part I: Forensic Medicine: Dedication , Preface , Introduction, Scope of Forensic Medicine, Aspects of Identification, Medico-legal Aspects of Death, Investigation of Death, Death by Asphyxia, Medico-legal Aspects of Injuries, Investigation of Wounds, Medico-legal Aspects of Sex Crimes, Medico-legal Aspects of Abortion, Forensic Pathology, Forensic Entomology, Radiation Poisoning, Medico-legal Sections in IPC, Cr PC, AND IE A, Part II: Toxicology: Introduction to Toxicology, General Approach to a Victim of Poison, Clinical Toxicology Laboratory, Practical Aspects of Analytical Toxicology, Toxicants of Public Health Hazard, Medical Toxicants, Environmental Toxicants, Abuse of Drugs, Natural Toxicants, Annexure I: Preparations of Reagents, Annexure II: Apparatuses, Annexure III: Glossary of Terms Used, Annexure IV: Abbreviations Used, Bibliography

Notes on Minor Surgery

By Dr. Debasish Kundu Ph.D. Guided & Edited by Dr. A.K. Banerjee M.B.B.S., M.D. (U.S.A.)

Rs. 395/- US $ 21.50 Paperback

CONTENTS: Part-I: Preface, Acharya Sushruta, Basic Surgical Procedures, Surgery of Some Common Conditions, Part II: Sterilisation, Suture Materials, Nomenclature of Operations, Planning for Operation, Anaesthesia,Operative Surgery, Postoperative Complications, Abscess Drainage, Venesection (Cut Down), Skin Grafting, Circumcision, Vasectomy, Hyderocele, Inguinal Hernia, Strangulated Inguinal Hernia, Femoral Hernia, Umbilical Hernia, Appendicetomy,

Abdominal Incisions, Peptic Ulcer, Vagotomy, Gastrojejumnostomy, Partial Gastrectomy, Closure of Perforated Peptic Ulcer, Right Hemicolectomy, Colostomy, Cholecystectomy, Choledocholithotomy (Supraduodenal), Spleenectomy, Lumbar Sympathectomy, Haemorrhoidectomy, Suprapubic Cystostomy, Prostatectomy, Exposure of Kidney , Exposure of the Ureter and Ureterolithotomy, Mastectomy, Thyroidectomy, Tracheostomy, Empyema Thoracis, Amputations, Bibliography

Principles and Practice of Naturopathy

By Dr. Debasish Kundu Editor Dr. Malik A. K. Awan Ph.D. (London) Associate Editor Prof. Sayed Farzin Hassanzadeh Salehian Ph.D.(Iran)

Rs. 750/- US $ 30.00 Paperback

CONTENTS: Foreword, Preface to the First Edition, Preface to the Third Edition, Naturopathy: Its Principles & Pioneers, Physiology, Food and Nutrition, Hygiene and Sanitation, Biology, Herbology, Medicinal Plants, Magnet Therapy, Yoga and Meditation, Massage Therapy, Medical Gymnastics, Chemistry, Bacteriology, Toxicology, Pathology, Osteology, Neurology, Ethics, Hydro Therapy and Helio Therapy, Colour Therapy, Fasting and Diet, Mud Therapy and Fango Therapy, Acupressure, Aromatherapy, Reflexology, Iridology, Vitamins and Balanced Diets, Bibliography

Diseases of Women (Adopted from Margaret Seifert's Krankheiten Der Franen)

By Dr. Shefalika Kundu, Edited By Dr. Debasish Kundu & Dr. Sudeshna Kundu

Rs. 350/- US $ 19.00 Paperback

The book is intended as a handbook on diseases of women with their Electrohomeopathic treatment. Besides an update on the literature on Contraception using Spagyrics , entirely new topics Anatomy of Uterus and Stages of development in Pregnancy are added.

CONTENTS: Preface to the Second Edition, Foreword to the First Edition, Preface, Introduction, Anatomy and Physiology of Sexual Organs of Women, General View of Treatment, Diseases and Their Treatment, Hygienic Care of the Body and Toilet, Anatomy of Uterus in Pregnancy, Notes on Various Diseases, Family Planning, Contraception in Electrohomoeopathy,Diet, Index of Diseases Discussed, Bibliography

Lectures on Materia Medica & Therapeutics

By Dr. H. D. Banerjee, Foreworded By M V Mattei, Thoroughly Revised & Edited By Prof. Dr. Debasish Kundu

Rs. 225/- US $ 18.00 Paperback

CONTENTS: Preface to the Third Edition, Preface to the Second Edition, Foreword to the First Edition, Introduction, On Electro-Homoeopathic Principles, On Principles of Orthodox School, On Homeopathic Principles , On Objections to Electro-Homoeopathy, Chemical Analysis of the Remedies, Dynamisation of the Remedies, On Minute Doses, On Frequency of the Doses, Purgatives in Electro-Homoeopathy, On Prescription Writing, Materia Medica & Therapeutics, On Therapeutics of the Remedies

Principles & Art of Cure in Electrohomeopathy

By Prof. Dr.Debasish Kundu Ph.D.

Rs. 195/- US $ 15.00 Paperback

CONTENTS: Introduction to Electrohomeopathy, Philosophy, The Discoverer, Principles of Nature, Introduction to Electrohomeopathy Medicines, The Iris science, Sources and preparation of Electrohomeopathy Medicines, Cohobation, Spagyric Tinctures, Classification of Electrohomeopathy Medicines, Classification, Preparation and Therapeutics uses of Electrohomeopathy Medicines, Potentisation of Electrohomeopathy Medicines and Electric fluids, Preparation and Therapeutic uses of Ointments and Lotions, Points for application Electric Fluids, Ointments and Lotions, Plain talks on using the medicines, Potentisation and Bio-Magnetism, The Similia of Electrohomeopathy, The Scientific basis of Electrohomeopathy System of Medicine, World's present day need of Electrohomeopathy, Clinical Index.

A Clinical Treatise on Cancer

By Prof. Dr.Debasish Kundu Ph.D. Foreworded By Dr. B.B. Upreti, Ph. D. General Secretary, All Nepal Electro-Homeo Medical Association, Hetauda, Nepal

Rs. 195/- US $ 15.00 Paperback

CONTENTS: Introduction, The Increase of Cancer and it's Causes, The Treatment of Cancer, Diet for Patients, Hygienic Care of the Patients

Books Published By LBO Publishing, 700 N Valley St., Suite B PMB 11884 Anaheim, CA 92801, USA Marketed In India Exclusively By Originals, Delhi

Pharmacodynamics in Spagyric Medicine(Plant Alchemy)

By Dr. Debasish Kundu & Dr.Sudeshna Kundu, Edited by Gisela Bruckel(Germany), El Akrem Hayouni (Tunisia), Forwarded by Dr.Peter Morrell (U.K.), Prof. Luigi Vernacchia & Dr.Fabio Ambrosi (Italy) Printed on Art Paper, USD ($) 70.00, Hardbound

It is the only trusted book to learn Sacred Alchemical Philosophy with Practical Laboratory Spagyrics, it covers from history & principles of Alchemy to the rarest topic Botanical Consciousness in Spagyrics, besides, Alchemy and the Zodiac Connection and how Spagyric Medicines work. In addition, detailed Pharmaceutical Process which are being carried out in most modern laboratories : from Apparatus, Vehicles, Sources of Medicines, Preparation of Spagyric Essences, quality control like Phytochemical Analysis, etc. , all major Spagyric Methods known to mankind, incl., Mattei, Zimpel, Junius, Solaris, Krauss,etc., besides the sacred Indian, Arabian and Chinese methods, Doctrine of Dosage, and much more. An Encyclopedia of Spagyrics or Plant Alchemy in one nutshell.

This work is edited by Gisela Bruckel, who is a Pharmacist and her Pharmacy in Wurzburg was the Main Dealer of Mattei Remedies in Europe till M V Mattei era, and Prof. El Akrem Hayouni, World famous authority on Plant Alchemy.

CONTENTS: Foreword, Preface, Part 1: Introduction to Spagyric Medicine, History of Alchemy, Principles of Spagyrics, The Simila of Alchemy, Difference Between Homoeopathy and Spagyric Homoeopathy, Botanical Consciousness in Spagyrics, Micronutrients and Spagyrics, Alchemy and the Zodiac Connection, How Spagyric Medicines Work, Alchemy and Spagyrics, Spagyrics : The Future in Medicine, Part 2: Pharmacy in Plant Alchemy, Pharmaceutical Process, Laboratory Apparatus, Vehicles Used in Plant Alchemy, Sources of Medicines, Preparation of Spagyric Essence, Spagyric Essence by Cohobation Method, Phytochemical Analysis of Plants, Different Spagyric Methods, Quality Control Procedures, Safety Measures in Laboratory, Doctrine of Dosage, Medicinal Plants, Terminology, Appendix, Bibliography

Mysticism, Romance & Secrets of Count Cesare Mattei (With Properly Transcripted Secret Formulas)

By Prof. Dr. Debasish Kundu , Ph.D. (U.S.A.)

Printed on Art Paper, USD ($) 40.00 Hard Bound

It is the Bible of Mattei Electrohomoeopathy : covering the true life of Cesare Mattei and properly transcripted Empirical Formulas & Secret Pharmacy of Electrohomoeopathy, incl. Medicinal Plants Used by Cesare Mattei.

Contributors-Prof. Raffaele Pezzani, University of Padova, Italy, Dr. Fabio R. Ambrosi, University of Sapienza, Rome, Italy, Prof. El Akrem Hayouni, University of Manouba, Tunisia, Allesandro Rapparini, Vice Pres., Archivio Museo Cesare Mattei, Bologna, Italy, Prof. Peter Morrell, Formerly Honorary Research Associate, History of Medicine, Staffordshire University, U.K., Dr. Terry Mitchell, Alchemist & Director, Phylak GmbH, U.K., Willow Morningsky, Spagyrist & Psychologist, Southern Oregon University, Ashland, Oregon, U.S.A. etc.

CONTENTS: Introduction, Dedication, Note to the Readers, Acknowledgements, Alchemist's Prayer, Preface, The Castle of Love, The Mystery Unveiled, Emerald Tablet of Cesare Mattei, Mysticism & Romance of Cesare Mattei, Electro Homoeopathy Pharmacology, Medicinal Plants Used by Cesare Mattei, Glossary of Pharmacological Terms, Bibliography

For Further Information and Ordering:
Originals/Low Price Publications
A-6, Second Floor, Nimri Commercial Centre,
Ashok Vihar Phase-4, Delhi - 110 052 (India)
Tel.: +91 11 2730 2453 Fax: 011 4706 1936
Mobile: 98100-12366
Website: www.Lppindia.com,
e-mail: info@Lppindia.com
info@Lbopub.com